Renal Diet Cookbook for Beginners

Face and Stop Your Kidney Disease Eating Healthier and Flavorfully. 201 Easy and Delicious Kidney-Friendly Recipes for a New Healthy Eating Style.

Lilian Nielsen

Table of Contents

INTRODUCTION

Human health depends on a complete balance when all of its interconnected bodily mechanisms function properly in perfect sync. If the major organs don´t work normally the body soon suffers indelible damage. Kidney malfunction is one such example, and it is not just the entire water balance that is disturbed by the kidney disease, but other diseases also emerge due to this problem. Kidney diseases are inherently progressive, meaning that if left unchecked and uncontrolled, they can ultimately lead to permanent kidney damage. That is why it is essential to control and manage the disease and put a halt to its progress, which can be done through medicinal and natural means. While medicines can guarantee only 30% of cure, a change of lifestyle and diet can prove to be miraculous with their 70% of guaranteed results. A kidney-friendly diet and lifestyle not only saves the kidneys from excess minerals but also aids medicines to work actively. Treatment without a good diet, hence, proves to be useless. In this renal diet cookbook, we shall bring out the basic facts about kidney diseases, their symptoms, causes, and diagnosis. This preliminary introduction can help the readers understand the problem clearly; then, we shall discuss the role of renal diet and kidney-friendly lifestyle in curbing the diseases. Moreover, the book also contains a range of delicious renal diet recipes that will guarantee luscious flavors and good health.

Despite their tiny size, the kidneys perform several functions that are vital for the body to be able to function healthily.

These include:

- Filtering excess fluids and waste from the blood.
- Creating the enzyme known as renin which regulates blood pressure.
- Ensuring bone marrow creates red blood cells.
- Controlling calcium and phosphorus levels through absorption and excretion.

Unfortunately, when kidney disease reaches a chronic stage, these functions start to stop working. However, with the right treatment and lifestyle, it is possible to manage symptoms and continue living well. This is even more applicable in the earlier stages of the disease.

Tactlessly, 10% of all adults over the age of 20 will experience some form of kidney disease in their lifetime. There are a variety of different treatments for kidney disease, which depend on the cause of the disease.

Kidney (or renal) diseases are affecting around 14% of the adult population according to international stats. In the US, approx. 661,000 Americans suffer from kidney dysfunction. Out of these patients, 468,000 proceed to dialysis treatment and the rest have one active kidney transplant.

The high quantities of diabetes and heart illness are additionally related to kidney dysfunction, and sometimes one condition, for example, diabetes, may prompt the other.

With such significant high rates, possibly the best course of treatment is the contravention of dialysis, which makes people depend upon clinical and crisis facility meds on any occasion multiple times every week. Thus, if your kidney has just given a few indications of brokenness, you can forestall dialysis through an eating routine, something that we will talk about in this book.

PART 1

Kidney Disease and Diet

CHAPTER 1

Understanding Kidney Disease

Kidney disease is becoming more prevalent in the United States, and so we need to learn as much about it as we can. The more we educate ourselves, the more we can do to take care of this important bodily system. If you've been diagnosed with chronic kidney disease (CKD), education can empower you to manage the disease more effectively and purposefully. Once you have a full understanding of what chronic kidney disease is, you can begin to take charge of your evolving health needs. Making healthy changes early in the stages of kidney disease will help you determine how to manage your kidney health. I am here to guide you, every step of the way. Like any new process, it may seem intimidating at first. But this chapter provides the foundation for learning and will help you to understand kidney disease as you begin your journey to healthier kidneys.

What Do the Kidneys Do?

Our kidneys are small, but they do powerful things to keep our bodies in balance. They are bean-shaped, about the size of a fist, and are located in the middle of the back, on the left and right sides of the spine, just below the rib cage. When everything is working properly, the kidneys do many important jobs such as:

- Filter waste materials from the blood.
- Remove extra fluid or water from the body.
- Release hormones that help manage blood pressure.
- Stimulate bone marrow to make red blood cells.
- Make an active form of vitamin D that promotes strong healthy bones.

What Causes Kidney Disease?

There are many causes of kidney disease, including physical injury or disorders that can damage the kidneys, but the two leading causes of kidney disease are diabetes and high blood pressure. These underlying conditions also put people at risk for developing cardiovascular disease. Early treatment may not only slow down the progression of the disease but also reduce your risk of developing heart disease or stroke.

Kidney disease can affect anyone, at any age. African Americans, Hispanics, and American Indians are at increased risk for kidney failure because these groups have a greater prevalence of diabetes and high blood pressure.

When we digest protein, our bodies create waste products. As blood flows through the capillaries, the waste products are filtered through the urine. Substances such as protein and red blood cells are too big to pass through the capillaries and so stay in the blood. All the extra work takes a toll on the kidneys. When kidney disease is detected in the early stages, several treatments may prevent the worsening of the disease. If kidney disease is detected in the later stages, high amounts of protein in your urine, called macroalbuminuria, can lead to end-stage renal disease.

High blood pressure, also known as hypertension; 1 of every 3 Americans is at risk for kidney disease because of hypertension. Although there is no cure for hypertension, certain medications, a low-sodium diet, and physical activity can lower blood pressure.

The kidneys help manage blood pressure, but when blood pressure is high, the heart has to work overtime at pumping blood. When the force of blood flow is high, blood vessels start to stretch so the blood can flow more easily. The stretching and scarring weaken the blood vessels throughout the entire body, including the kidneys. And when the kidneys' blood vessels are injured, they may not remove the waste and extra fluid from the body, creating a dangerous cycle, because the extra fluid in the blood vessels can increase blood pressure even more.

With diabetes, excess blood sugar remains in the bloodstream. The high blood sugar levels can damage the blood vessels in the kidneys and elsewhere in the body. And since high blood pressure is a complication from diabetes, the extra pressure can weaken the walls of the blood vessels, which can lead to a heart attack or stroke.

Other conditions, such as drug abuse and certain autoimmune diseases, can also cause injury to the kidneys. In fact, every drug we put into our body has to pass through the kidneys for filtration.

An autoimmune disease is one in which the immune system, designed to protect the body from illness, sees the body as an invader and attacks its own systems, including the kidneys. Some forms of lupus, for example, attack the kidneys. Another autoimmune disease that can lead to kidney failure is Goodpasture´s Syndrome, a group of conditions that affect the kidneys and the lungs. The damage to the kidneys from autoimmune diseases can lead to chronic kidney disease and kidney failure.

Treatment Plans for Chronic Kidney Disease (CKD)

The best way to manage CKD is to be an active participant in your treatment program, regardless of your stage of renal disease. Proper treatment involves a combination of working with a healthcare team, adhering to a renal diet, and making healthy lifestyle decisions. These can all have a profoundly positive effect on your kidney disease—especially watching how you eat.

Working With Your Healthcare Team

When you have kidney disease, working in partnership with your healthcare team can be extremely important in your treatment program, as well as being personally empowering. Regularly meeting with your physician or healthcare team can give you resources and information that help you to make informed decisions regarding your treatment needs, and provide you with a necessary opportunity to vent, share information, get advice, and receive support in effectively managing this illness.

Adhering to a Renal Diet

The heart of this book is the renal diet. Sticking to this diet can make a huge difference in your health and vitality. Like any change, following the diet may not be easy at first. Important changes to your diet, particularly early on, can prevent the need for dialysis. These changes include limiting salt, eating a low-protein diet, reducing fat intake, and getting enough calories if you need to lose weight. Be honest with yourself first and foremost—learn what you need, and consider your personal goals and obstacles. Start by making small changes. It is okay to have some slip-ups—we all do. With guidance and support, these small changes will become habits of your promising new lifestyle. Immediately, you will begin taking control of your diet and health.

Making Healthy Lifestyle Decisions

Lifestyle choices play a crucial part in our health, especially when it comes to helping regulate kidney disease. Lifestyle choices such as allotting time for physical activity, getting enough sleep, managing weight, reducing stress, and limiting smoking and alcohol will help you take control of your overall health, making it easier to manage your kidney disease. Follow this simple formula: Keep toxins out of your body as much as you can, and build up your immune system with a good balance of exercise, relaxation, and sleep.

CHAPTER 2

The Causes of Renal Failure

Renal disease, according to experts, requires early diagnosis and targeted treatment to prevent or delay both a condition of acute or chronic renal failure and the appearance of cardiovascular complications to which it is often associated.

In fact, hypertension and diabetes, not adequately controlled by drug therapy, prostatic hypertrophy, kidney stones or bulky tumors can promote onset as they reduce the normal flow of urine, increase the pressure inside the kidneys and limit functionality.

Or the kidney damage can be determined by inflammatory processes (pyelonephritis, glomerulonephritis), or by the formation of cysts inside the kidneys (polycystic kidney disease), or by the chronic use of some drugs, alcohol, and drugs consumed in excess.

A fundamental role in alleviating the work of the already compromised kidneys is carried out by the diet which is, therefore, the first prevention. It must be studied with a nutrient expert per serving or a nephrologist, to maintain or reach an ideal weight on the one hand, and the other to reduce the intake of sodium (salt), the consequent control of blood pressure, and/or other substances (minerals), without creating malnutrition or nutritional deficiencies. Particular attention should also be paid to cholesterol, triglycerides, and blood sugar levels.

Understanding what causes kidney failure goes a long way to deciding just what kind of treatment you should focus on. The most important factor that you should focus on is, of course, your diet. But as you focus on your diet, make sure that you are following your doctor's instructions, in the event of other complications. Let us look at a few of the common causes of kidney diseases.

Diabetes

We do know that diabetes is one of the leading causes of CKD. But we have yet to understand in detail why and how it can cause so much harm to the kidneys.
Time for a crash course in diabetes. What many may already know is that diabetes affects our body's insulin production rate. But what many may not know is the extent of damage that diabetes can cause to the kidneys.

High Blood Pressure

An important thing to remember here is that high blood pressure can be both a cause and symptom of CKD, similar to the case of diabetes.
So, what exactly is blood pressure? People often throw the term around, but they are unable to pinpoint exactly what happens when the pressure in the blood increases.

Autoimmune Diseases

IgA nephropathy and lupus are two examples of autoimmune diseases that can lead to kidney diseases. But just what exactly are autoimmune diseases?
They are conditions where your immune system perceives your body as a threat and begins to attack it.
We all know that the immune system is like the defense force of our body. It is responsible for guiding the soldiers of our body, known as white blood cells, or WBCs. The immune system is responsible for fighting against foreign materials, such as viruses and bacteria. When the system senses these foreign bodies, various fighter cells, including the WBCs, are deployed to combat the threat.

Typically, your immune system is a self-learning system. This means that it is capable of understanding the threat and memorizing its features, behaviors, and attack patterns. This is an important capability of the immune system since it allows the system to differentiate between our cells and foreign cells. But when you have an autoimmune disease, your immune system suddenly considers certain parts of your body, such as your skin or joints, as foreign. It then proceeds to create antibodies that begin to combat as a threat that parts of your body, which can result in damages to important organs like your kidneys.

Symptoms of Kidney Disease?

If kidney disease progresses, then the blood level of end products of metabolism increases; this, in turn, is the cause of feeling unwell. Various health problems may occur, such as high blood pressure, anemia, bone disease, premature cardiovascular calcification, discoloration, and change in the composition and volume of urine.

As the disease progresses, the main symptoms can be:

- Weakness, a feeling of weakness
- Trouble sleeping
- Lack of appetite
- Dry skin, itchy skin
- Muscle cramps especially at night
- Swelling in the legs
- Swelling around the eyes, especially in the morning

Diagnose With Kidney Disease

There are two simple tests that your family doctor can prescribe to diagnose kidney disease.

Blood Test: Glomerular Filtration Rate (GFR) and Serum Creatinine Level

Creatinine is one of those end products of protein metabolism, the level of which in the blood depends on age, gender, muscle mass, nutrition, physical activity, the foods taken before taking the sample (for example, a lot of meat was eaten), and some drugs. Creatinine is removed from the body through the kidneys, and if the work of the kidneys slows down, the level of creatinine in the blood plasma increases. Determining the level of creatinine alone is not sufficient for the diagnosis of chronic kidney disease since its value begins to exceed the upper limit of the norm only when GFR is decreased by half. GFR is calculated using a formula that includes 4 parameters which are: the creatinine reading, age, gender, and race of the patient. GFR shows the level at which the kidneys can filter. In the case of chronic kidney disease, the GFR indicator indicates the stage of the severity of kidney disease.

Urine Analysis

The content of albumin in the urine is determined by the analysis; also, the values of albumin and creatinine in the urine are determined by each other. Albumin is a protein that usually enters the urine in minimal quantities. Even a small increase in the level of albumin in the urine for some people may be an early sign of incipient kidney disease, especially in those with diabetes and high blood pressure. In the case of normal kidney function, albumin in the urine should not be more than 3 mg./mmol (or 30 mg./g.). If albumin excretion increases even more, then it already speaks of kidney disease.

CHAPTER 3

Stages of Kidney Disease

According to the National Kidney Foundation in the US, kidney disease can be classified into 5 different progressive stages. These stages and their symptoms do not only help the doctor to devise an appropriate therapy but also guide the patient to take the necessary measures in routine life. The rate of kidney function tells much about these phases. In the early stages, there is minimum loss of function, and this loss increases with every stage.

The eGFR is used as a standard criterion to measure kidney function. The acronym eGFR means estimated Glomerular Filtration Rate. It is the rate at which the waste material is transferred from the blood to the nephron's tubes through the "glomerulus"—the filtering membrane of the kidney tissues. The lesser the rate of glomerular filtration, the greater the problem the kidneys are going through. A person's age, gender, race, and serum creatinine are entered into a mathematical formula to calculate their eGFR. The serum creatinine level is measured in a blood test. The creatinine is a waste product of the body which is produced out of muscular activities. Healthy kidneys are capable of removing all the creatinine out of the blood. A rising creatinine level is therefore a sign of kidney disease. It is said that if a person has been having an eGFR of less than 60 for 3 months, it means that they are suffering from serious renal problems.

The 5 main stages of chronic kidney disease can be categorized as follows:

Stage 1

The first stage starts when the eGFR gets slightly higher than the normal value. In this stage, the eGFR can be equal to or greater than 90 ml./min.

Stage 2

The next stage arises when the eGFR starts to decline and ranges between 60–89 ml./min. It is best to control the progression of the disease at this point.

Stage 3

From this point on, the kidney disease becomes concerning for the patient as the eGFR drops to 30–59 ml./min. At this stage, consultation is essential for the health of the patient.

Stage 4

Stage 4 is also known as Severe Chronic Kidney Disease as the eGFR level drops to 15–29 ml./min.

Stage 5

The final and most critical phase of chronic renal disease is stage 5, where the estimated glomerular filtration rate gets as low as below 15 ml./min.

Role of Potassium, Sodium, and Phosphorus

Sodium

Sodium is considered the most important electrolyte of the body next to chloride and potassium. The electrolytes are the substance that controls the flow of fluids in and out of the cells. Sodium is mainly responsible for regulating blood volume and pressure. It is also involved in controlling muscle contraction and nerve functions. The acid-base balance in the blood and other body fluids is also regulated by sodium. Though sodium is important for the health and regulation of important body mechanisms, excessive sodium intake, especially when a person suffers from some stages of chronic kidney disease, can be dangerous. Excess sodium disrupts the critical fluid balance in the body and inside the kidneys. It then leads to high blood pressure, which in turn negatively affects the kidneys. Salt is one of the major sources of sodium in our diet, and it is strictly forbidden on the renal diet. High sodium intake can also lead to edema, which is swelling of the face, hands, and legs. Furthermore, high blood pressure can stress the heart and cause the weakening of its muscles. The build-up of fluid in the lungs also leads to shortness of breath.

Potassium

Potassium is another mineral that is closely linked to renal health. Potassium is another important electrolyte, so it maintains the fluid balance in the body and its pH levels as well. This electrolyte also plays an important role in controlling nerve impulses and muscular activity. It works in conjugation with the sodium to carry out all these functions. The normal potassium level in the blood must range between 3.5 and 5.5 mEq/L. It is the kidneys that help maintain this balance, but without their proper function, the potassium starts to buildup in the blood. Hyperkalemia is a condition characterized by high potassium levels. It usually occurs in people with chronic kidney disease. The prominent symptoms of high potassium are numbness, slow pulse rate, weakness, and nausea. Potassium is present in green vegetables and some fruits, and these ingredients should be avoided on a renal diet.

Phosphorus

The amount of phosphorus in the blood is largely linked to the functioning of the kidneys. Phosphorus, in combination with vitamin D, calcium, and parathyroid hormone, can regulate renal function. The balance of phosphorus and calcium is maintained by the kidneys, and this balance keeps the bones and teeth healthy. Phosphorus, along with vitamin D, ensures the absorption of calcium into the bones and teeth, where this mineral is important for the body. On the other hand, it gets dangerous when the kidneys fail to control the amount of phosphorus in the blood. This may lead to heart and bone-related problems. Mainly there is a high risk of weakening of the bones followed by the hardening of the tissues due to the deposition of phosphorus and calcium outside the bones. This abnormal calcification can occur in the lungs, skin, joints, and arteries, which can become in time very painful. It may also result in bone pain and itching.

CHAPTER 4

How to Limit Sodium, Potassium, and Phosphorus in the Diet

Limit the Sodium, Phosphorus, Potassium, and Calcium

Sodium is found in many foods; it is more than only table salt. It is important to be careful with this mineral and your consumption of it, especially when you have high blood pressure or chronic kidney disease. This is because sodium affects the water balance in your body and can greatly raise your blood pressure in the process, causing more kidney damage and increasing your risk of heart disease. Thankfully, your doctor can run a simple blood test to see the mineral levels in your bloodstream, which will allow you to know whether or not your sodium levels are too high.

If your blood pressure is at a healthy level, and you are only in the early stages of chronic kidney disease, you can aim for 2–3 g. of sodium a day. However, if you are in the later stages of kidney disease with high blood pressure, you should reduce your sodium consumption to below 2 g. daily.

To cut your sodium consumption, you should avoid:

- Table salt
- Sea salt
- Garlic salt
- Seasoning salt
- Soy sauce
- Onion salt
- Celery salt
- Meat tenderizer

- Lemon pepper
- Oyster sauce
- Teriyaki sauce
- Barbecue sauce
- Cured foods, such as meats and vegetables
- Lunch meats

Most fast foods and highly processed foods are high in sodium, meaning that cooking at home is your best option. This doesn't mean you have to cook difficult and elaborate meals; they can be simple and easy. Since you cannot include salt, instead enjoy a wide selection of sodium-free spices and herbs. Whenever you cook with canned foods, you should drain off the liquid and then rinse the food in warm water, to remove excess sodium. Lastly, always read ingredient labels to check the sodium content.

It is important to watch your phosphorus levels, to prevent a buildup in your bloodstream. Ask your doctor how much phosphorus you should aim for as your daily intake. In general, when a person develops late-stage kidney disease, their doctor will advise them to consume no more than one gram of phosphorus daily.
You can limit your phosphorus intake by limiting dairy consumption, cutting back on meats and fish, reading ingredient and nutrition labels to avoid high phosphorus ingredients, avoiding dark-colored sodas, increasing fresh fruits and vegetables, and consuming more rice and corn products.

Your doctor will likely recommend that you reduce your calcium intake, which shouldn't be difficult as foods high in calcium are generally also high in phosphorus. This means you naturally will not be consuming much calcium. The easiest way to reduce your calcium intake is to limit dairy products, bone-in fish, seeds, and fortified foods.

Lastly, you should limit your potassium intake. This mineral is really important, but most people consume much more than they need. While this is not generally a problem, it becomes one for people with decreased renal function as their kidneys are no longer able to filter out the excess potassium, causing a buildup in the bloodstream. This can be more difficult to avoid, as many foods are rich in potassium, such as fruits and vegetables. In general, you don't want to consume any more than 2 g. of potassium daily.

Try to limit potassium-rich foods, such as:

- Tomatoes
- Potatoes
- Sweet potatoes
- Cranberries
- Blueberries
- Strawberries
- Raspberries

- Plums
- Star fruit
- Avocados
- Bananas
- Whole-wheat bread
- Brown rice
- Dairy
- Oranges
- Apricots
- Winter squash
- Beets
- Dark leafy greens
- Dried fruits
- Parsnips
- Rutabaga

Kidney Disease Diet for Stage 5 and Dialysis Patients

When you are in the fifth stage of chronic kidney disease, in which your kidneys fail and you most likely begin dialysis, you have to take even more precautions than you do in stages 1–4 of kidney disease. This means that you have to be even more careful in which foods you eat, how much protein you consume, and the number of minerals in your meals.

Since you will now be on dialysis, you will need to limit your fluid and food intake that causes a buildup of waste or excess minerals in the bloodstream. Your doctor, renal dietitian, and the dialysis center should be able to help you monitor your diet and answer any questions you might need. These doctors, dietitians, and nurses are there to help and can help you customize your diet to ideally fit your needs.

If you also have high blood pressure, high cholesterol, or diabetes, you will be happy to know that this diet will not only benefit your chronic kidney disease but your other conditions, as well.

In general, dialysis patients need to:

- Consume more protein-rich foods.
- Consume less sodium, phosphorus, and potassium.
- Control fluid intake including water, tea, coffee, juices, and other beverages.

Fluids

While many people in today's day and age do not drink enough water, the same is not true of dialysis patients. People who are undergoing dialysis therapy can easily consume too much water, causing a fluid overload known as hypervolemia. The kidneys are responsible for balancing the amount of fluid in your body, but when this is disrupted is can negatively affect your health, causing swelling and difficulty breathing.

When a person begins dialysis treatment, their kidneys are no longer able to balance the amount of fluid in the body. This results in them being unable to remove enough fluid, causing a buildup in the body. This is also why you have to be even more vigilant in reducing sodium intake, as sodium affects your body's fluid levels. Thankfully, if you can carefully manage both your fluid and sodium intake, your dialysis treatments should be able to maintain the correct amount of these in your body, removing any excess.

If you are worried you may have consumed too much liquid you should watch for symptoms of swelling in your hands, feet, and face; shortness of breath; high blood pressure; cramping, headaches, and bloating; and heart problems such as changes in your heart rate or palpitations. You can better manage your fluid intake by tracking how much you are drinking. Some people may prefer to do this with a small notebook they can keep on them, although it is generally easier to use a smartphone app. There are many apps designed to track your liquid intake. Remember, when tracking your intake don't only track water, but all the liquid you consume. You can better manage your thirst by sucking on sugar-free hard candies, frozen grapes, and ice chips. These can help you to avoid drinking too much between your dialysis therapy sessions.

Keep in mind that sodium causes your body to hold onto water. You will have to be even more careful with your sodium intake than you were in earlier stages of kidney disease.
Follow the fluid recommendations given to you by your doctor and dialysis team. This will vary from person to person based on their body and various lifestyle factors. However, most people are instructed to limit their fluid intake to only 32 oz. daily.
If you have concerns about developing fluid overload, then talk with your healthcare team. They may need to adjust your dialysis treatments to account for any concerns, such as including either longer or more frequent dialysis treatments.

Meat and Protein

While people in earlier stages of kidney disease need to limit their protein intake, patients in stage 5 who are on dialysis will be required to increase their protein intake. By increasing your protein, you can maintain healthy blood protein levels and improve your overall health. Try choosing fish, poultry, and eggs while generally avoiding red meat, which is high in saturated fats. In general, you will want to eat 8–10 oz. of high-protein ingredients, such as meat, dairy.
Beans, lentils, peas, nuts, seeds, and peanuts will have to be eaten in moderation. Keep in mind that these foods are high in phosphorus and potassium, so you should only eat small servings of them when it does not cause you to go over your daily limit.

Grains and Cereals

Grains and cereals can be a great option, in some cases. Not everyone can enjoy these foods as if you are having trouble managing your blood sugar; they could spike it even more. Therefore, it is generally best for diabetic patients to limit grains.

When choosing grains try to avoid whole-grain or high-fiber varieties, such as brown rice and whole-wheat bread. While these are generally better options for healthy people, the same is not true for those with chronic kidney disease, as they contain a larger amount of phosphorus. Instead, choose the processed forms of grains such as white rice, pasta, and white bread.

Fruits and Vegetables

When consuming fruits and vegetables, you want to select varieties that are low in phosphorus and potassium. It is helpful that canned fruits are lower in potassium than fresh alternates. On the other hand, canned vegetables have more sodium and should be rinsed off before being consumed.
It is a good idea to download a diet app on your smartphone and track what you eat. Try to find an app option that will give you the full nutritional details of what you are eating, so that you can easily track your mineral intake and reduce the risk of overconsumption.

Try to consume 23 servings of low-potassium fruits daily, such as:

-
- 1 apple
- 5 pears
- 1 peach
- 1 tangerine
- 2 plums
- 10 cherries
- 5 cup berries
- 5 cups fruit cocktail, drained
- 15 grapes
- 5 cup pineapple, canned, drained
- 1 watermelon, small wedge

Consume 2–3 servings of low-potassium vegetables daily. Keep in mind that they will all have some potassium, which you need to track so that you aren't consuming more than you believe.

Some options include:

- Cabbage
- Radishes
- Broccoli
- String beans
- Lettuce
- Eggplant
- Celery
- Watercress
- Peppers
- Cauliflower
- Carrots
- Eggplant
- Yellow squash
- Zucchini
- Onions

CHAPTER 5

Benefits of Renal Diet

If you have been diagnosed with kidney dysfunction, a proper diet is necessary for controlling the amount of toxic waste in the bloodstream. When toxic waste piles up in the system along with increased fluid, chronic inflammation occurs and we have a much higher chance of developing cardiovascular, bone, metabolic, or other health issues.

Since your kidneys can't fully get rid of the waste on their own, which comes from food and drinks, probably the only natural way to help our system is through this diet.

Benefits

A renal diet is especially useful during the first stages of kidney dysfunction and leads to the following benefits:

- Prevents excess fluid and waste buildup.
- Prevents the progression of renal dysfunction stages.
- Decreases the likelihood of developing other chronic health problems e.g. heart disorders.
- Has a mild antioxidant function in the body, which keeps inflammation and inflammatory responses under control.

The above-mentioned benefits are noticeable once the patient follows the diet for at least a month and then continuing it for longer periods, to avoid the stage where dialysis is needed. The strictness of the diet depends on the current stage of renal/kidney disease, if, for example, you are in stage 3 or 4, you should follow a stricter diet and be attentive to the food, which is allowed or prohibited.

These exact foods and nutrients that you should take when following a renal diet, will be given to you in the following sections, and so keep on reading.

Explanation of Key Diet Words

The following nutrients play a major role in a renal diet as some can improve the condition while others can make it worse. Essentially, a renal diet is based on low consumption of certain nutrients like potassium and phosphorus simply because it promotes fluid buildup within the system of a kidney patient. Here is a brief explanation of the function of each nutrient and its role in a renal diet:

Potassium

Potassium is a mineral that naturally occurs in certain foods and plays a role in regulating heart rhythm and muscle movement. It is also needed for keeping fluid and electrolyte balance at normal levels. Our kidneys keep only the right levels of potassium in our system, and when it is excess, they expel it via the urine.

The problem is, once kidneys can't function properly, all this excess potassium can't be expelled out and spikes up, causing symptoms like muscle and bone weakness, abnormal heartbeat, and heart failure in extreme cases.

Thus, a diet low in potassium is recommended to prevent buildup and avoid such negative side effects.

Sodium

Sodium is a trace mineral that is found in most foods that we eat today and it is the key component of salt, which is a sodium compound mixed with chloride. Most food that we consume and specially processed food is highly loaded with salt, however, we may be eating sodium in other forms too e.g. fish. The key role of sodium is to regulate blood pressure, help regulate nerve function, and maintain the balance of acids in the blood. However, when sodium is excessively high and the kidneys can expel it, it can lead to the following symptoms: an elevated feeling of thirst, swelling of hands, feet, and face, elevated blood pressure, and problems with breathing.

This is why it is suggested to keep sodium intake low, to avoid the above.

Phosphorus

Phosphorus is an essential mineral that is responsible for the development and regeneration of our bones. Phosphorus also plays a key role in the growth of connective tissue e.g. muscles and the regulation of muscle motions. When the food we take contains phosphorus, it gets absorbed by the intestines and then gets deposited in our bones.

However, when kidneys are damaged or dysfunctioning, the excess phosphorus can't be expelled through our systems and causes problems such as: extracting calcium out of the bones/making them weaker, and leading to excess calcium in the bloodstream which interferes with blood vessels, heart, eye, and lung function.

Protein

Protein is a nutritional compound that consists of amino acids, which play a key role in various system functions like cell communication, oxygen supply, and cellular metabolism. They are also a part of a healthy immune system.

Normally, protein is not an issue for our kidneys. When protein is metabolized, waste by-products are also created and are filtered through the kidneys. This waste along with extra-renal proteins will be expelled through urine.

However, when kidneys are unable to filter out excess protein, it gets accumulated in the blood and cause problems.

This doesn't mean that renal disease patients should avoid protein totally as it is still necessary for some metabolic functions, as long as it's taken in moderate amounts and based on the stage of renal disease.

Carbohydrates

Carb act as a key source of fuel for our bodies. The consumption of carb is turned into glucose in our system, which is a primary source of energy.

Carbs are ok to be eaten in moderation by kidney patients and the daily recommended allowance is up to 150 g./day. However, patients that also suffer from diabetes (besides renal disease) should control their carb consumption to avoid any sudden spikes in their blood glucose.

Fats

Being in balanced amounts, fats in our bodies act as an energy source, aid in the release of hormones, and help regulate blood pressure. They also carry some vitamins that are fat-soluble such as A, D, E, and K, which are also very important for our systems. Not all fats are created equal though, some are good for our health and some are bad. Bad fats are saturated and trans fats, founded in processed meat, dairy, and other products. They are also found in margarine and vegetable fat shortenings.

Fats, in general, don't pose a risk for renal disease patients, however, it is suggested to limit the consumption of saturated and trans fats to avoid any cardiovascular problems e.g. elevated blood pressure and clogging of the arteries.

Dietary fiber

Dietary fiber is a compound that can't be digested on its own by enzymes and acids in our stomach and intestines but is needed for the system to aid in the digestion of our food and encourage bowel movements. They generally promote bowel regularity and decrease the likelihood of developing constipation inside the colon. Dietary fiber is typically found in fruits, vegetables, seeds, and whole grains.

In patients with renal disease, dietary fiber is ok up to 28 g./day as long as these plant foods don't contain high amounts of phosphorus or potassium.

Vitamins

According to medical and dietary guidelines, our bodies need close to 13 vitamins to functions. Vitamins play a key role in metabolic functions and the normal functioning of our cardiovascular, digestive, nervous system, and immune systems. The adoption of a nutritionally dense and balanced diet is necessary for getting all the vitamins our system needs. However, due to some diet restrictions e.g. sodium, many renal patients need water-soluble vitamins like B-complex (B1, B2, B6, B12, folic acid, biotin) and small amounts of Vitamin C.

Minerals

Minerals are needed for our system to maintain healthy connective tissue e.g. bones, muscles, and skin, and facilitate the normal function of our hearts and central nervous systems.

Our kidneys typically expel any excess amount of minerals through urine as some can lead to health symptoms e.g. muscle spasms when their levels are abnormally high.

However, as it was mentioned earlier, some minerals like potassium and phosphorus cannot be expelled by our kidneys when are in excess, so their intake through diet should be limited. Other trace minerals are perfectly fine when following a renal diet: iron, copper, zinc, and selenium. A lack of these can lead to increased oxidative stress, thus, is important to take sufficient amounts through diet or supplementation.

Fluids

Fluids are necessary for the proper hydration of our systems in fact; lack of fluids can lead to dehydration and death in extreme cases.

However, in patients with renal dysfunction, fluids can quickly buildup to the point of placing pressure on vital organs like the lungs and heart and becoming dangerous. This is the reason why many physicians advise their kidney patients to limit the consumption of fluids, especially during the last stages of the disorder.

Managing Kidney Disease Through Diet

Patients who struggle with kidney health issues, going through kidney dialysis, and have renal impairments need to not only go through medical treatment but also change their eating habits and lifestyle to make the situation better. Many types of research have been done on this, and the conclusion is food has a lot to do with how your kidney functions and its overall health.

The first thing to changing your lifestyle is knowing about how your kidney functions and how different food can trigger different reactions in the kidney function. Certain nutrients affect your kidney directly. Nutrients like sodium, protein, phosphate, and potassium are the risky ones. You do not have to omit them altogether from your diet, but you need to limit or minimize their intake as much as possible. You cannot leave out essential nutrients like protein from your diet, but you need to count how much protein you are having per day. This is essential to keep balance in your muscles and maintaining a good functioning kidney.

A vast change in kidney patients is measuring how much fluid they are drinking. This is a crucial change in every kidney patient, and you must adapt to this new eating habit. Too much water or any other form of liquid can disrupt your kidney function. How much fluid you can consume depends on the condition of your kidney. Most people assign separate bottles for them so that they can measure how much they have drunk, and how much more they can drink throughout the day.

CHAPTER 6

What You Can Eat, What to Avoid

Foods You Need

Many foods work well within the renal diet, and once you see the available variety, it will not seem as restrictive or difficult to follow. The key is focusing on the foods with a high level of nutrients, which make it easier for the kidneys to process waste by not adding too much that the body needs to discard. Balance is a major factor in maintaining and improving long-term renal function.

Garlic

Garlic is an excellent, vitamin-rich food for the immune system and a tasty substitute for salt in a variety of dishes. It acts as a significant source of vitamin C and B6 while aiding the kidneys in ridding the body of unwanted toxins. It's a great, healthy way to add flavor to skillet meals, pasta, soups, and stews.

Berries

All berries are considered a good renal diet food due to their high level of fiber, antioxidants, and delicious taste, making them an easy option to include as a light snack or as an ingredient in smoothies, salads, and light desserts. Just one handful of blueberries can provide almost one day's vitamin C requirement, as well as a boost of fiber, which is good for weight loss and maintenance.

Bell Peppers

Flavorful and easy to enjoy both raw and cooked, bell peppers offer a good source of vitamin C, vitamin A, and fiber. Along with other kidney-friendly foods, they make the detoxification process much easier while boosting your body's nutrient level to prevent further health conditions and reduce existing deficiencies.

Onions

This nutritious and tasty vegetable is excellent as a companion to garlic in many dishes, or on its own. Like garlic, onions can provide flavor as an alternative to salt, and provides a good source of vitamin C, vitamin B, manganese, and fiber, as well. Adding just one quarter or half of the onion is often enough for most meals, because of its strong, pungent flavor.

Macadamia Nuts

If you enjoy nuts and seeds as snacks, you may soon learn that many contain high amounts of phosphorus and should be avoided or limited as much as possible. Fortunately, macadamia nuts are an easier option to digest and process, as they contain much lower amounts of phosphorus and make an excellent substitute for other nuts. They are a good source of other nutrients, as well, such as vitamin B, copper, manganese, iron, and healthy fats.

Pineapple

Unlike other fruits that are high in potassium, pineapple is an option that can be enjoyed more often than bananas and kiwis. Citrus fruits are generally high in potassium as well, so if you find yourself craving an orange or grapefruit, choose pineapple instead. In addition to providing high levels of vitamin B and fiber, pineapples can reduce inflammation thanks to an enzyme called bromelain.

Mushrooms

In general, mushrooms are a safe, healthy option for the renal diet, especially the shiitake variety, which are high in nutrients such as selenium, vitamin B, and manganese. They contain a moderate amount of plant-based protein, which is easier for your body to digest and use than animal proteins. Shiitake and Portobello mushrooms are often used in vegan diets as a meat substitute, due to their texture and pleasant flavor.

Foods You Need to Avoid

Eating restrictions might be different depending upon your level of kidney disease. If you are in the early stages of kidney disease, you may have different restrictions as compared to those who are at the end-stage renal disease, or kidney failure. In contrast to this, people with an end-stage renal disease requiring dialysis will face different eating restrictions. Let's discuss some of the foods to avoid while being on the renal diet.

Dark-Colored Colas

They contain calories, sugar, phosphorus, etc. They contain phosphorus to enhance flavor, increase their life, and avoid discoloration. Which can be found in a product's ingredient list. This addition of phosphorus varies depending on the type of cola. Mostly, the dark-colored colas contain 50–100 mg. in 200 ml. serving. Therefore, dark colas should be avoided on a renal diet.

Canned Foods

This includes soups, vegetables, and beans, which are low in cost but contain high amounts of sodium due to the addition of salt to increase its life. Is better that people with kidney disease should avoid consumption. Opt for lower-sodium content with the label "no salt added". One more way is to drain or rinse canned foods, such as canned beans and tuna, which could decrease the sodium content by 33–80%, depending on the product.

Brown Rice

This is a whole grain containing a higher concentration of potassium and phosphorus than its white rice counterpart. A cooked brown rice cup contains about 150 mg. of phosphorus and 154 mg. of potassium, whereas, one cup of already cooked white rice has an amount of about 69 mg. of phosphorus and 54 mg. of potassium. Bulgur, buckwheat, pearled barley, and couscous are equally beneficial, low-phosphorus options and might be a good alternative instead of brown rice.

Bananas

Bananas are high potassium content, low in sodium, and provides 422 mg. of potassium per banana. It might disturb your daily balanced potassium intake to 2,000 mg. if a banana is a daily staple.

Whole-Wheat Bread

This bread may harm individuals with kidney disease, but for healthy individuals it is ok. White bread is recommended for individuals with kidney disease just because it has phosphorus and potassium. But if you add more bran and whole grains to the bread, then the amount of phosphorus and potassium contents goes higher.

Oranges and Orange Juice

These are enriched with vitamin C content and potassium. 184 g. provides 333 mg. of potassium and 473 mg. of potassium in one cup of orange juice. With these calculations, oranges and orange juice must be avoided or used in a limited amount while being on a renal diet.

Potatoes and Sweet Potatoes

These are potassium-rich vegetables. 156 g. of potatoes contains 610 mg. of potassium, whereas 114 g. of sweet potatoes contains 541 mg. of potassium which is relatively high. Some of the high-potassium foods, likewise potatoes and sweet potatoes, could also be soaked or leached to lessen the concentration of potassium contents. Cut them into small and thin pieces and boil those for at least 10 minutes can reduce the potassium content by about 50%. Potatoes soaked in a wide pot of water for at least 4 hours before cooking could possess even less potassium content than those not soaked before cooking. This is known as "potassium leaching," or the "double cook direction."

If you are suffering from or living with kidney disease, reducing your potassium, phosphorus, and sodium intake is an essential aspect of managing and tackling the disease. The foods with high-potassium, high-sodium, and high-phosphorus content listed above should always be limited or avoided. These restrictions and nutrients intakes may differ depending on the level of damage to your kidneys. Following a renal diet might be a daunting procedure and restrictive most times. But, working with your physician, nutrition specialist, and a renal dietitian can help you to formulate a renal diet specific to your individual needs.

CHAPTER 7

Stage by Stage Nutritional Needs

A Kidney-Friendly Lifestyle

Once a kidney is damaged there is no one-time solution or magic to undo all the damage. It requires constant management and a whole new lifestyle to provide a healthy environment for your kidneys. For healthy kidneys, you just need to keep the following in mind:

- Upgrade your vegetable intake to 5–9 vegetables per day.
- Reduce the salt intake in your diet.
- Cut down the overall protein intake.
- Remove all the triggers of heart diseases, like fats and sugar, from your diet.
- Do not consume pesticides and other environmental contaminants.
- Try to consume fresh food; homemade is the best.
- Avoid using food additives, as they contain high amounts of potassium, sodium, and phosphorus.
- Drink lots of sodium-free drinks, especially water.
- Choose to be more active and exercise regularly.
- Do not smoke to avoid toxicity.
- Obesity can create a greater risk of kidney diseases, so control your weight.
- Do not take painkillers excessively, such as ibuprofen, as they can also damage your kidneys.

Kitchen Staples

Spices and Herbs

- Oregano
- Thyme
- Onion powder
- Garlic powder
- Paprika
- Cayenne pepper
- Black pepper
- Chili powder
- Cumin
- Basil
- Rosemary

Vegetables

- Onions
- Garlic
- Carrots
- Celery
- Bell peppers
- Green beans
- Wild rice
- Beets
- Cucumbers
- Peas

Fruits

- Apples
- Pineapples
- Blueberries
- Strawberries
- Raspberries
- Cranberries
- Bananas

Meat and Poultry

- Pork chops
- Beef briskets
- Chicken legs
- Chicken breasts
- Turkey breasts
- Oysters

Dairy

- Eggs
- Yogurt
- Cheese
- Low-fat milk
- Rice milk

Miscellaneous

- Chia seeds
- Farfel
- Flour
- Sesame seeds (black and white)
- Sesame oil
- Olive oil
- Cherry pie filling
- Pie crusts
- Butter
- Sweet sauce
- Hot sauce
- Splenda
- Oyster crackers
- Tortilla
- Low sodium bouillon cubes

CHAPTER 8

Frequently Asked Questions

Q1. How Can We Avoid Phosphate Additives in our Kidney Diet?

The practice of reading the labels can save you from all the trouble. It is not just the phosphates but a great number of other ingredients detrimental to a good renal diet that you can identify this way. When phosphate additives are present in the food, the label usually contains the E sign followed by a number showing the type of phosphate added to the product. Here is a list of commonly present phosphates in additives.

- E339 Sodium phosphates
- E338 Phosphoric acid
- E340 Potassium phosphates
- E343 Magnesium phosphates
- E545 Ammonium polyphosphates
- E450 Triphosphates
- E542 Bone phosphate
- E341 Calcium phosphates
- E540 Calcium phosphate
- E541 Sodium aluminum phosphate
- E544 Calcium polyphosphates

Q2. What are the Suitable Alternatives to Salt?

No spice and seasoning can indeed replace salt, but when health comes first we can make a little compromise on taste and try something that can infuse delicious flavors into our food even though not exactly like salt. Down below are a few examples that can be used to season beef, fish, pork, chicken and stews, etc.

- For beef, you can use dry mustard, allspice, bay leaf, oregano, chili powder, and cayenne pepper.
- For the seasoning of the fish, you can use lemon, vinegar, mint, dill, thyme, chili, garlic.
- To spice up the pork, you can use apple sauce, cloves, garlic powder, sage, onion powder, curry powder.
- When it comes to chicken and turkey, you can always use garlic, lemon, rosemary, thyme, chili powder, tarragon, sage, cayenne pepper, and paprika to season the meat.
- For stews and casseroles, try some sage, oregano, basil, thyme, and garlic to add flavors.

Q3. Is It Safe to Take Herbal Supplements on the Renal Diet?

Herbal supplements may contain some of the minerals that can be harmful to renal patients. There is a certain level of risk involved in the intake of these supplements without consulting a doctor and/or dietician. If you have been taking these supplements, ask your doctor if you should continue their use. Discuss it in detail with your medical care provider and ask for their approval. If they contain kidney damaging substances, then it is best to avoid them altogether. You can always take other supplements suitable for the renal diet.

Q4. What if a Person Has Multiple Medical Conditions, How Can They Make this Diet Fit for All?

It is recommended to always consult a health expert and a dietician first and let them check your medical conditions. Based on the diagnosis, the dietician will create a suitable diet formula to fit all your medical conditions. Proper diagnosis is essential before adopting this renal diet.

Q5. Is It True that Soaking Potatoes Releases Their Excess Potassium?

There are primarily 2 ways to remove potassium from potatoes. Soaking the potatoes in water is one such method. The other is a double boiling method. The latter is far more effective than the former when it comes to the removal of potassium. The simple soaking does work effectively. Therefore, it is recommended to soak the potato slices into hot boiled water and leave it until it cools down, then replace it with another round of hot water, then drain to use the potatoes. The second method is to boil the potatoes in water until they turn soft. It is important to remember here that the potatoes must be peeled and diced before they are added to the boiling water. These 2 methods can reduce the potassium in the potatoes down to 50% of its original percentage. So, potato lovers are suggested to make use of these methods and enjoy potatoes as they please.

Q6. Can We Use Artificial Sweeteners on the Renal Diet?

Yes, there are many artificial sweeteners that are not prohibited on the renal diet. Stevia, sugar alcohols, aspartame, saccharin, and sucralose are some of the artificial sweeteners which can be freely used on the renal diet, as they do not contain any harmful additives. But it is always important to check the source and authenticity of the products you are using. It is best to consult your dietician and ask about the specific product you want to use.

Q7. How to Deal With Low Appetite Problems in CKD?

When a person suffers from renal disease, they automatically lose their appetite. It is largely because of the fluid, electrolytes, and hormonal imbalance in the body. But despite this lowering of appetite, it is important for a person to meet their caloric and protein needs to avoid malnutrition. There are a few measures you can take to overcome this problem.

- Try to consume small yet frequent meals in a day. Eat something healthy after 2–3 hours.
- Always take the full meal when you feel the best of your appetite. It is ok if you don't feel like eating at the exact time of lunch, dinner, or breakfast.
- If you go out for work or some other engagements, it is best to carry some healthy snacks along with you. Eat bits of your snack every 2 hours.
- Set an alarm or a reminder on your cellphone according to the meal and snack time and try to follow that schedule.
- Try to add more variety to the food and add more flavors and colors to your platter. The more exciting and tempting your food will be, the better your appetite will get.
- Do more physical activities to elevate your metabolism rate and digestion. Take a brisk walk or do some light exercise in this regard.
- You can also ask your health expert to recommend some kidney-friendly supplements to meet the energy and protein needs of your body.
- It does not matter how much you eat; what is important is the nutritional quality of the food you are eating. Keep that in mind every time to eat something.

CHAPTER 9

Food List for the Renal Diet

Phosphorus

This mineral can be found in every cell of our bodies, but mostly in the teeth and bones—it provides structural support to DNA and RNA. Phosphorus also helps us filter waste from the kidneys, but interestingly, too much phosphorus can be detrimental in CKD. Healthy kidneys can filter excess phosphorus and other waste from the body, but during early-stage kidney disease, the kidneys must work harder to remove it. Studies reveal that reducing phosphorus intake in earlier stages of CKD may help maintain kidney function as well as healthy bones and a healthy heart.

For people with CKD and those receiving dialysis, phosphorus in the diet should be restricted to between 800 and 1,000 mg. per day. Talk with your dietitian or healthcare provider, who can tell you if you need to limit foods that are high in phosphorus, and/or prescribe a phosphate binder to help control your phosphorus levels.

Phosphorus in Common Foods*

LOW PHOSPHORUS (Less than 150 mg./serving)	MEDIUM PHOSPHORUS (151–250 mg./serving)	HIGH PHOSPHORUS (More than 251 mg./serving)
Apple	Beans, black, 1 cup	Peanuts, oil roasted, 2 oz.
Bagel, 1 plain (4-inch diameter)	Beans, fava, 1 cup	Almonds, oil/dry roasted, 2 oz.
Barley, pearled, cooked	Beans, kidney, 1 cup	Baked beans, 1 cup
Beans, green	Beans, pinto, 1 cup	Beans, small white, mature, boiled, 1 cup

Bread, pita, 1 (6.5-inch diameter)	Beef, bottom round, 3 oz.	Beef, liver, cooked, 3 oz.
Bread, pumpernickel, 2 slices	Beef, chuck roast, 3 oz.	Beefalo, 3 oz.
Bread, white, 2 slices	Beef, eye round, 3 oz.	Buttermilk, 1 cup
Butter, 1 tbsp.	Beef, ground, 70% lean, 3 oz.	Calamari, fried, 3 oz.
Cabbage	Beef, ground, 95% lean, 3 oz.	Cashews, dry roasted, 2 oz.
Cauliflower	Beef, sirloin steak, 3 oz.	Cereal, bran, 100%
Cereal, crispy rice, 1 cup	Black-eyed peas, 1 cup	Cereal, wheat germ, 1/4 cup
Cheese, Brie, 1 oz.	Bread, whole wheat, 2 slices	Cheese, goat, 2 oz.
Cheese, feta, 1 oz.	Catfish, breaded/fried, 3 oz.	Cheese, Parmesan, 2 oz.
Cocoa, unsweetened, 2 tbsp.	Cheese, blue, 2 oz.	Cheese, ricotta, part-skim
Cookies, shortbread, 4	Cheese, Cheddar, 1 oz.	Cheese, Romano, 2 oz.
Cornflakes, 1 cup	Cheese, mozzarella, 1 oz.	Chia seeds, 1 oz.
Cottage cheese, nonfat	Cheese, provolone, 2 oz.	Chicken, liver, cooked, 3 oz.
Couscous, cooked	Cheese, Swiss, 1 oz.	Clam chowder, New England
Cream cheese, 1 oz.	Chicken, breast, 3 oz.	Clams, cooked with moist heat, 3 oz.
Cucumber	Chicken, dark meat, 3 oz.	Cornbread, 1 piece
Duck, with skin, 3 oz.	Chickpeas, 1 cup	Crab, Alaska king, cooked with moist heat, 3 oz.
Egg white, 1 large	Chocolate, plain, 2 oz.	Custard, flan, 1 cup
Egg yolk, 1 large	Cod, Pacific, 3 oz.	Flounder, 3 oz.
Eggplant	Cottage cheese, 1% fat	Halibut, Atlantic/Pacific, 3 oz.
English muffin, 1 plain	Cottage cheese, 2% fat	Lentils, mature, boiled, 1 cup
Figs	Crab, blue, cooked with moist heat, 3 oz.	Milk, 1%, 1 cup
Gelatin, water base	Crab, Dungeness, cooked with moist heat, 3 oz.	Milk, chocolate, 1 cup
Ginger ale, 1 can	Lamb, kabobs, domestic, 3 oz.	Milk, evaporated, nonfat
Grapefruit	Lamb, leg roast, domestic, 3 oz.	Milk, nonfat, 1 cup
Grapes	Lamb, New Zealand, 3 oz.	Milk, whole, 1 cup
Grouper	Lobster, cooked with moist heat, 3 oz.	Mussels, blue, cooked with moist heat, 3 oz.
Hominy grits	Macadamia nuts, 3 oz.	Nuts, Brazil, 2 oz.

Ice cream, 10% fat, vanilla	Milk, canned, sweetened, condensed, 1/4 cup	Nuts, pine, 2 oz.
Lettuce	Mushrooms, cooked, 1 cup	Oysters, Eastern, cooked with moist heat, 3 oz.
Milk, soy, 1 cup	Mussels, raw, blue, 3 oz.	Peanuts, boiled, 1 cup
Oatmeal, cooked, 1 packet	Peanut butter, 2 tbsp.	Peanuts, dry roasted, 3 oz.
Onions	Pork, boneless loin chop, 3 oz.	Peanuts, oil/roasted, 2 oz.
Oysters, canned, 3 oz.	Pork, leg roast, 3 oz.	Pecans, oil/dry roasted, 3 oz.
Oysters, raw, Pacific, 3 oz.	Raisin Bran, 1 cup	Salmon, canned, pink/red, 3 oz.
Pasta, 1 cup	Raisins, seedless, 1 cup	Sardines, canned in oil, 3 oz.
Peas, split, mature, boiled	Rice, brown, cooked, 1 cup	Scallops, breaded/fried, 3 oz.
Plums	Shredded Wheat, 1 cup	Sole, 3 oz.
Popcorn, air-popped, 1 cup	Shrimp, breaded/fried, 3 oz.	Soybeans, mature, boiled
Pork, spare ribs, 3 oz.	Snapper, 3 oz.	Sunflower seeds, 1 oz.
Radishes	Spinach, raw	Swordfish, 3 oz.
Rice cakes, 1 cake	Tortilla, 2 corn or flour (6-inch diameter)	Tofu, raw, firm
Rice, white, enriched, cooked	Turkey, breast, 3 oz.	Tuna, light, canned in oil, 3 oz.
Sherbet	Turkey, dark meat, 3 oz.	Tuna, white, canned in oil, 3 oz.
Shrimp, cooked with moist heat, 3 oz.	Veal, rib roast, 3 oz.	Veal, cubed, stewed, 3 oz.
Sour cream	Wheat flakes, 1 cup	Walnuts, English, 2 oz.
Tofu, soft		Wheat flour, whole grain, 1 cup
Wheat flour, white, 1 cup		Yogurt, low-fat
		Yogurt, skim
* One serving = 1/2 cup unless otherwise noted.		

Protein

Protein plays an important role in the body and is crucial to staying healthy. It allows your body to counteract everyday wear and tear, heal from injury, stop bleeding, and fight infections. However, too much protein can put a strain on your kidneys, and even cause additional damage. You can talk with your healthcare provider about how a reduced protein diet may help slow the progression of CKD. If you're in the early stages of chronic kidney disease, such as stages 1 and 2, your protein intake will be limited to 12–15% of your calorie intake each day, which is the same level recommended by the Dietary Reference Intakes (DRIs) for a healthy diet for normal adults. For example, if you are following a 2,000-calorie diet, your protein intake should be limited to 60–75 g. of protein (see Calculate Your Intake, here). People receiving dialysis should take in about 1.2 g. of protein per kg. of body weight each day (1 kg. is about 2.2 lb.). For those in stages 3 and 4, recommended protein intake is between 0.6 and 0.75 g./kg, according to the Kidney Disease Outcomes Quality Initiative (KDOQI) of The National Kidney Foundation.

As you choose your protein sources, it's important to know that some foods contain more useful and healthy proteins than others.

Sodium

Sodium is an important mineral that helps regulate your body's water content and blood pressure. Sodium is also a major electrolyte, which helps control the fluid in the body's tissues and cells. When your kidneys are working the way they are supposed to, they can remove sodium from the body as needed. However, much like phosphorus, when your kidneys are not working properly the sodium build up in your body and make your blood pressure rise, make you thirsty, and result in water retention, causing you to gain weight.

For people in the early stages of chronic kidney disease—stages 1, 2, or 3—it is suggested that you restrict your sodium intake to between 2,000 mg. and 3,000 mg. per day (see Calculate Your Intake, above). If you have stage 4 or 5 chronic kidney disease and require dialysis, even lower amounts may be prescribed. It is suggested that you ingest no more than 1,500 mg. of sodium each day.

Potassium

Potassium is a mineral and electrolyte that regulates metabolism and fluid levels and helps your muscles, kidneys, and heart function properly, but only in the right doses—it depends on how well your kidneys are working and whether you are taking medications that affect potassium levels. In the early stages of kidney disease, potassium levels are usually normal. If your potassium level is above normal during stages 1, 2, or 3 of CKD, your physician will probably conduct a blood test to help determine the cause and whether you need to make any dietary changes.

Potassium in Common Foods*

LOW POTASSIUM	MEDIUM POTASSIUM (151–250 mg./serving)	HIGH POTASSIUM
(Less than 150 mg./serving)	Apple, without skin, 1 large	(More than 251 mg./serving)
Alfalfa seeds, sprouted, raw	Apricot, halves, 1 medium	Apricot, 1 cup
Apple juice	Apricots, in a heavy syrup, drained	Artichoke, 1 medium
Applesauce, sweetened	Asparagus, boiled, 5 spears	Avocado
Bagel, 1 plain (4-inch diameter)	Beans, green, boiled, 1 cup	Bamboo shoots, cooked
Beans, green, frozen	Blackberries, 1 cup	Banana, 1 small
Blueberries	Broccoli, frozen, 1 cup	Beans, black, mature, boiled
Cabbage, shredded, boiled	Brussels sprouts, boiled	Beans, dried
Carrot, baby raw, 1 medium	Carrots, sliced, 1 cup	Beans, lima, large, mature, boiled, 1/3 cup
Cherries, sour canned, in syrup	Cereal, All-Bran	Beans, pinto, mature, boiled
Coffee, 1 cup	Cherries, 10 sweet	Beans, refried, canned
Cranberries, dried	Chickpeas, dried, boiled	Beets, cooked
Cranberry juice	Collards, chopped, frozen	Cabbage, Chinese, cooked
Cranberry sauce, canned	Corn, yellow, boiled, 1 ear	Cantaloupe, cubed, 1 cup
Eggplant, boiled	Date, dried, 1 date	Chard, Swiss, boiled, 1/3 cup
Fig, raw, 1 medium	Elderberries	Chocolate
Ginger ale, 12 oz.	Grapefruit, 1/2 medium	Dates, Medjool
Grapes	Grapefruit juice	Fruits, dried
Lemon, 1 medium	Grape juice, 1 cup	Mango, pieces, 1 cup
Lime, 1 medium	Honeydew melon, pieces	Milk, 1%, 1 cup
Mustard greens, frozen	Kiwifruit, 1 medium	Milk, soy, 1 cup
Oatmeal, regular	Leeks, 1 raw	Milk, whole, 1 cup
Okra, cooked	Mustard greens, cooked, 3/4 cup	Molasses, 1 tbsp.
Onions, raw, diced	Onion, chopped, boiled	Mushrooms, cooked, 1 cup
Parsley, raw, 10 sprigs	Orange, 1 medium	Nectarine, 1 medium
Peaches, canned, in syrup, drained	Peach, 1 small	Nuts, mixed, 2 oz.

Pears, canned, in syrup, drained	Pear, 1 medium	Orange juice, fresh
Peppers, sweet, cooked	Peppers, hot chili	Papaya, 1 small
Pineapple, pieces	Peppers, sweet, raw	Plantain, sliced, cooked
Plum, 1 medium	Pineapple, canned	Pomegranate, 1 small
Popcorn, buttered	Pineapple juice	Pomegranate juice
Prunes, dried, 1 prune	Prickly pear, 1 medium	Potatoes, white, baked, 1 medium
Radicchio, raw, shredded	Prunes, canned, 5 prunes	Raisins, seedless, 1.5-oz. box
Raspberries	Radishes, raw, sliced, 1 cup	Sapodilla, 1 medium
Rhubarb, cooked with sugar	Raspberries, frozen, sweetened, 1 cup	Sauerkraut, undrained, 1 cup
Rice, white, enriched, 1 cup cooked	Scallions, chopped, raw, 1 cup	Spinach, cooked
Spaghetti, enriched, cooked	Squash, summer	Succotash, boiled
Spinach, raw, chopped	Strawberries, whole, 1 cup	Sweet potatoes, boiled
Tea, black, 8 oz.	Tangerine, 1 large	Tomato, 1 medium
Turnips, white, cubed	Tortillas, corn, 4 (6-inch diameter)	Tomato paste, canned, 1/4 cup
Water chestnuts, canned	Turnip greens, chopped	Tomato sauce, canned, 1/4 cup
Watermelon, pieces	* One serving = 1/2 cup unless otherwise noted.	Water chestnuts, raw
* One serving = 1/2 cup unless otherwise noted.		

CHAPTER 10

2-Week Meal Plan

Day 1

- Breakfast: Turkey and spinach scramble on melba toast
- Lunch: Lasagna spaghetti squash
- Snack: 2 Cranberry orange cookies
- Dinner: Thai fish soup

Day 2

- Breakfast: Cornbread with southern twist
- Lunch: Spiced honey salmon
- Snack: 1 serving roasted mint carrots
- Dinner: Roasted sirloin steak

Day 3

- Breakfast: Cherry-pineapple bread
- Lunch: Light paprika moussaka
- Snack: Walnut butter on a cracker (1 serving = 2 crackers)
- Dinner: Seafood corn chowder

Day 4

- Breakfast: Baked egg muffins
- Lunch: Chickpea curry
- Snack: 1 serving date & blueberry muffins
- Dinner: Laurel lamb

Day 5

- Breakfast: Cheese spaghetti frittata
- Lunch: Herbed vegetable trout
- Snack: 1 serving savory collard chips
- Dinner: Creamy turkey

Day 6

- Breakfast: Strawberry topped waffles
- Lunch: Easy pork kebab
- Snack: 2 choco-chip cookies
- Dinner: Fiery jalapeño poppers

Day 7

- Breakfast: French toast with apple sauce
- Lunch: Grilled lemon cod
- Snack: Creamy dandelion greens and smoothie

- Dinner: Beef with red kidney beans

Day 8

- Breakfast: Strawberry & blueberry muesli
- Lunch: Mixed pepper paella
- Snack: 1 serving Chocolate coconut quinoa slices
- Dinner: Citrus glazed salmon

Day 9

- Breakfast: Grandma's pancakes special
- Lunch: Beef patties
- Snack: Cinnamon apple chips
- Dinner: Broccoli cheese pie

Day 10

- Breakfast: Pasta with Indian lentils
- Lunch: Broiled shrimps
- Snack: Almond & Blueberry smoothie
- Dinner: Cabbage borscht

Day 11

- Breakfast: Parmesan zucchini frittata
- Lunch: Asparagus pasta
- Snack: 1 serving Spiced pumpkin pancake
- Dinner: Lemon pepper chicken legs

Day 12

- Breakfast: Garlic mayo bread
- Lunch: Stuffed bell peppers with quinoa
- Snack: Pineapple raspberry parfait
- Dinner: Feta lamb patties

Day 13

- Breakfast: Shrimp bruschetta
- Lunch: Almond pasta salad
- Snack: Almonds & zucchini smoothie
- Dinner: Turkey broccoli salad

Day 14

- Breakfast: Bagels made healthy + 1 tbsp. walnut butter
- Lunch: Shredded beef
- Snack: 2 choco-chip cookies
- Dinner: Curried onion and cauliflower soup

Tips

Tips on Controlling Your Phosphorus

Here is what you should do to maintain a balanced level of phosphorus:

- Limit the consumption of foods like poultry, meats, fish, and dairy.
- Limit the intake of certain dairy products like yogurt and cheese; you should not exceed 4 oz. per serving.
- Avoid black beans, lima beans, red beans, garbanzo beans, white beans, and black-eyed peas.
- Avoid unrefined, whole, and dark grains.
- Stay away from refrigerator dough.
- Avoid dried fruits and vegetables.
- Avoid chocolate.

- Avoid dark-colored sodas.
- Make sure to take your phosphate folders with your snacks and meals.
- The renal diet limits the intake of phosphorus to 1,000 mg. per day.

Tips on Controlling Your Protein

- Make sure to consume high-quality proteins. Eat about 7–8 oz. of protein per day. Pork, beef, turkey, veal; chicken, and eggs have high amounts of protein.

Tips on Controlling Your Fluid Intake

- Use 1 cup or glass to divide your fluid intake per day. You can also write a record of your fluid intake.
- Always avoid any type of salty food and never add extra salt to your meals.
- Avoid processed meats, fast foods, and canned foods.
- You can add lemon juice to the water you want to drink instead.
- You can clean your mouth with a mouthwash from time to time.
- Avoid overheating.
- Maintain your blood sugar at a balanced level.
- Extra tip to reduce potassium of potatoes: place potatoes in a pot with warm water for soaking for about 3–4 hours. Dry well before cooking.

Eating Out

Look out for small or half portions, and ask your server for your foods to be cooked without extra salt, butter, or sauce. Avoid fried foods, instead, embrace poached or grilled food. If you know, you are going out to eat, plan ahead. Look at the restaurant menu beforehand online.

Eating at Social Gatherings (Such as Birthdays, Weddings, Picnics, and Barbecues)

- Don't go hungry: Have a snack before you leave the house.
- Avoid high-sodium foods: Avoid foods such as hot dogs or sausages. Choose lower-sodium foods such as chicken and hamburgers.
- Limit alcohol: Speak with your physician first about drinking alcohol.
- Plan ahead: Plan your menus.

Shopping List

Vegetables

-
- Eggplant
- Endive
- Ginger root
- Lettuce
- Onions
- Parsley
- Radishes
- Spaghetti squash
- Turnips
- Vegetables, mixed
- Water chestnuts, canned
- Bread and cereals
- Cereals, Kellogg's Corn Flakes
- Cereals, Cheerios
- Cereals, Corn Chex

Beverages

- 7UP
- Coffee
- Cream soda
- Fruit punch
- Ginger ale
- Grape soda
- Hi-C
- Lemon-lime soda
- Lemonade
- Orange soda
- Root beer
- Tea
- Dairy and dairy alternatives
- Almond milk
- Coffee-mate
- Rich's Coffee Rich

Other

- Apple butter
- Sugar, brown or white
- Sugar, powdered

Time-Saving Strategies

If you are always on the go, with errands to run, dinner to make, and a schedule to maintain, grocery shopping can test your patience.

Keep yourself on track with these 6 tips for efficient food shopping:

- Don't shop on an empty stomach. Go shopping after you've eaten. This will help you avoid buying unhealthy food products.
- Have your shopping list ready. Keep your grocery list organized and efficient, arranging items by category or grouping items that are usually found in the same aisle. There are two advantages to this trick: you spend less time in the grocery store, and you are less likely to forget something.
- Plan ahead. Try to plan out your meals and foods for the week. It will save you time, and you won't stress out over daily menu planning.
- Keep it simple. Your shopping trip doesn't have to be time-consuming. Do you have coffee, sugar, cereal, bread, fruit, or milk? What will you be packing for lunch? Do you have the recipe, so you can jot down the ingredients you need ahead of time?
- Fresh is best. One of the best places to grocery shop is at your local farmers' market.

Farmers' markets always have the freshest and most delicious produce. When you consider the value of organic, local foods, and their potential positive effect on your health, you won't mind paying a little more at the farmers' market.

Eating healthy and maintaining a kidney-friendly diet doesn't have to be hard. With the right amount of planning, a little prep work, and a good grocery-store strategy, creating a healthy meal plan can be easy and fun.

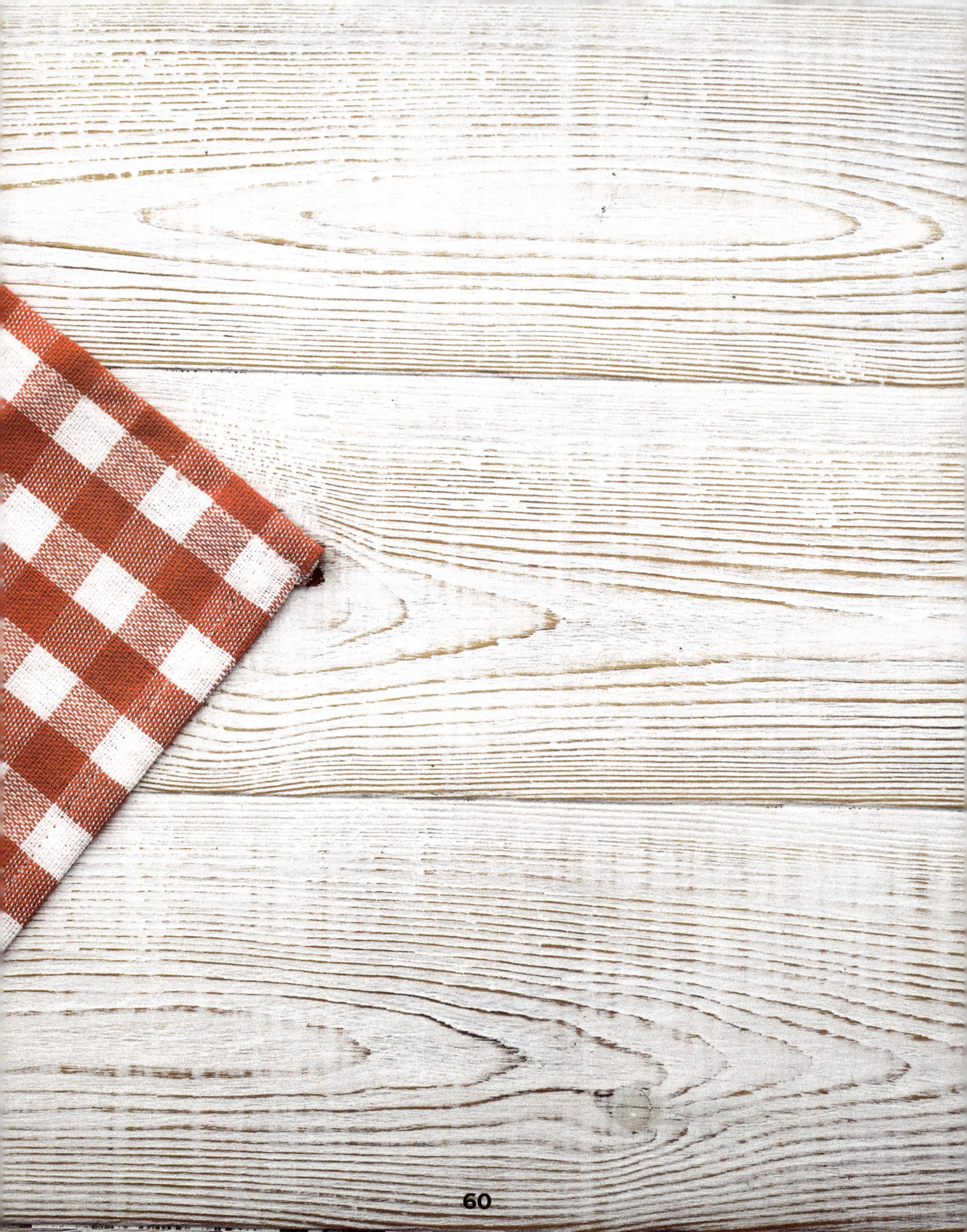

PART 2

Kidney - Friendly Recipes

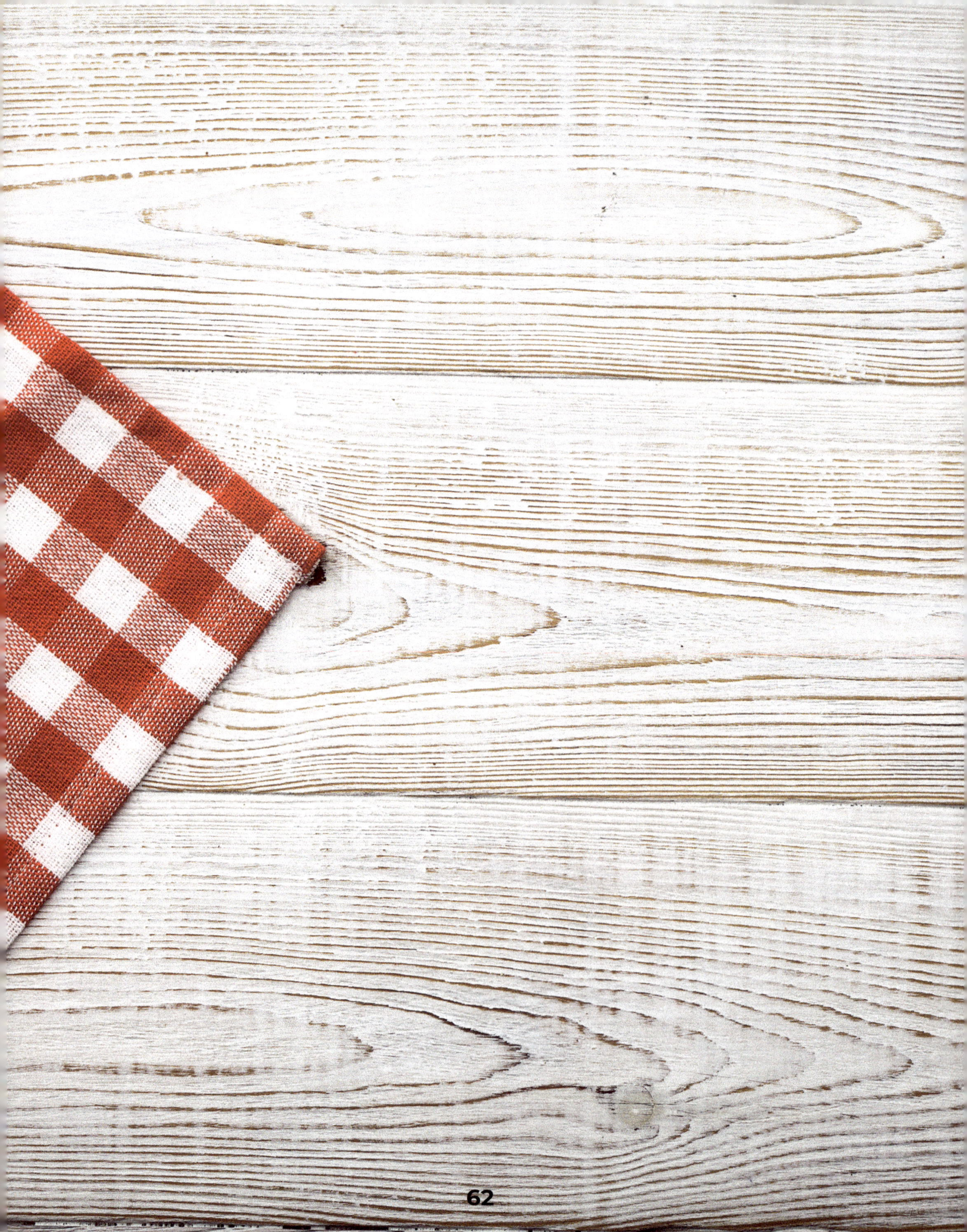

CHAPTER 11

Breakfast and Brunch

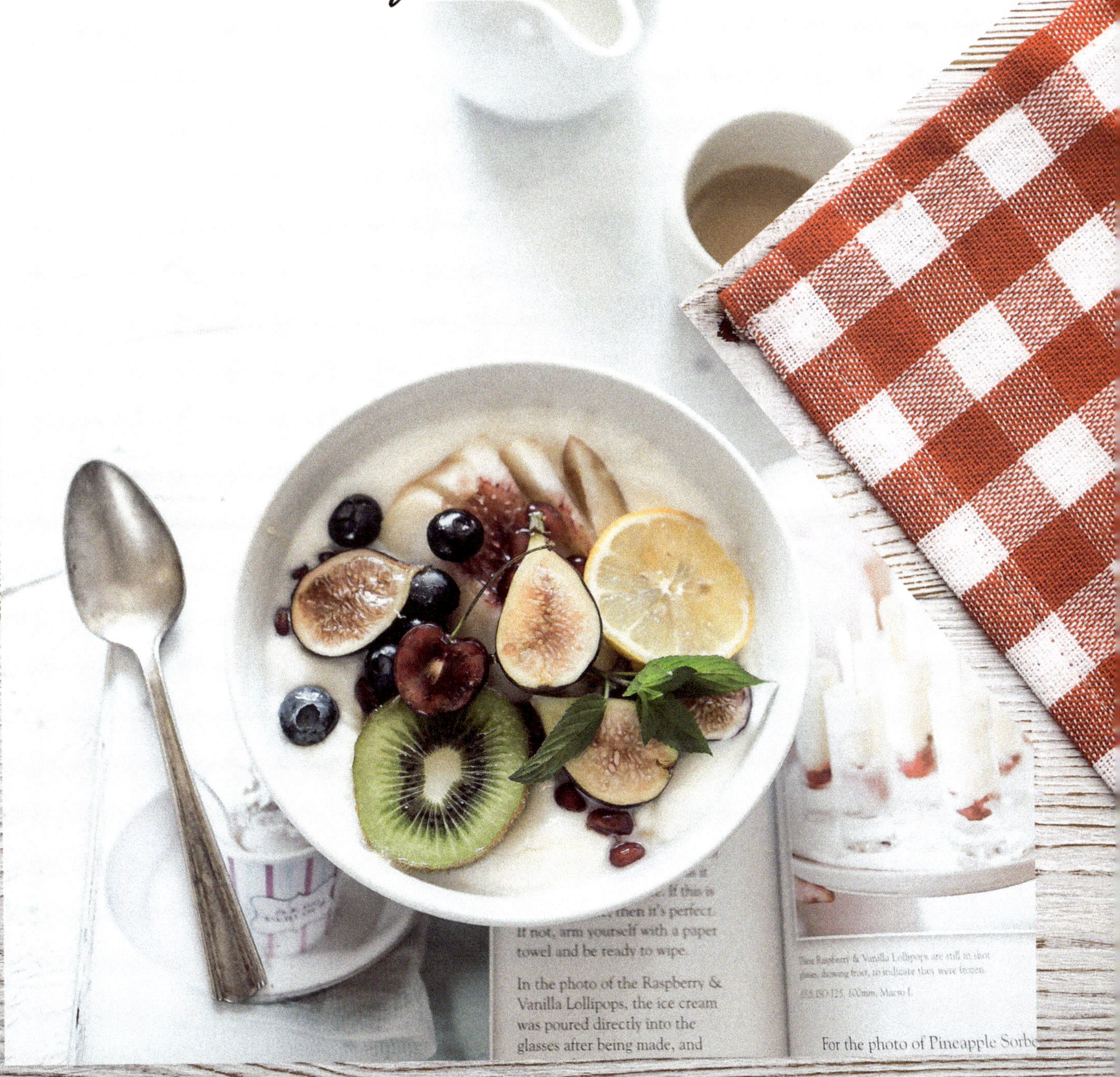

1. Turkey and Spinach Scramble on Melba Toast

PREPARATION TIME
3'

COOK TIME
15'

SERVING
4

INGREDIENTS

- 1 tsp. extra virgin olive oil
- 1 cup turkey breast, cooked and diced
- 1 cup raw spinach
- 1/2 garlic clove, minced
- 1 tsp. nutmeg, grated or dried
- 4 slices melba toast
- 1 tsp. balsamic vinegar

DIRECTIONS

1. Heat a skillet on medium heat and add oil.
2. Add your turkey pieces to the pan and heat through for 6–8 minutes.
3. Now add the spinach, garlic, and nutmeg and allow to cook for a further 6 minutes, stirring now and then to prevent the garlic from browning.
4. Plate up the melba toast and top with the spinach and turkey scramble.
5. Drizzle with a little balsamic vinegar if desired and serve.

NUTRIENTS PER SERVING

- Calories: 88
- Protein 12 g.
- Fat: 2 g.
- Carb: 5 g.
- Sodium: 56 mg.
- Potassium: 170 mg.
- Phosphorus: 102 mg.

2. French Toast With Applesauce

PREPARATION TIME
5'

COOK TIME
15'

SERVING
2

INGREDIENTS

- 3/4 cup unsweetened applesauce
- 1/2 cup milk
- 1 tsp. ground cinnamon
- 2 eggs
- 4 slices whole-wheat bread

DIRECTIONS

1. Mix well applesauce, cinnamon, milk, and eggs in a mixing bowl.
2. Soak the bread, one by one into an applesauce mixture until wet.
3. On medium fire, heat a nonstick skillet greased with cooking spray.
4. Add soaked bread one at a time and cook for 2–3 minutes per side or until lightly browned.
5. Serve and enjoy.

NUTRIENTS PER SERVING

- Calories: 352
- Protein: 12 g.
- Fat: 8 g.
- Carb: 60 g.
- Sodium: 462 mg.
- Potassium 254 mg.
- Phosphorus 184 mg.

3. Bagels Made Healthy

PREPARATION TIME
5'

COOK TIME
25'

SERVING
8

INGREDIENTS

- 2 tsp. yeast
- 1 1/2 tbsp. olive oil
- 1 1/4 cups bread flour
- 2 cups whole-wheat flour
- 1 tbsp. vinegar
- 2 tbsp. honey
- 1 1/2 cups warm water

DIRECTIONS

1. In a bread machine, mix all ingredients, and then process on dough cycle.
2. Once done or end of the cycle, create 8 pieces shaped like a flattened ball.
3. In the center of each ball, make a hole using your thumb then create a donut shape.
4. In a greased baking sheet, place donut-shaped dough then covers and let it rise about 1/2 hour.
5. Prepare about 2 inches of water to boil in a large pan.
6. In boiling water, drop one at a time the bagels and boil for 1 minute, then turn them once.
7. Remove them and return them to a baking sheet and bake at 350°F (175°C) for about 20–25 minutes until golden brown.

NUTRIENTS PER SERVING

- Calories: 221
- Protein 7 g.
- Carb: 42 g.
- Protein: 7 g.
- Sodium 47 mg.
- Potassium 166 mg.
- Phosphorus: 130 mg.

4. Cornbread With Southern Twist

PREPARATION TIME
15'

COOK TIME
60'

SERVING
8

INGREDIENTS

- 2 tbsp. shortening
- 1 1/4 cups skim milk
- 1/4 cup egg
- 4 tbsp. sodium-free baking powder
- 1/2 cup flour
- 1 1/2 cups cornmeal

DIRECTIONS

1. Prepare an 8x8-inch baking dish or a black iron skillet then add shortening.
2. Put the baking dish or skillet inside the oven at 425°F, once the shortening has melted that means the pan is hot already.
3. In a bowl, add milk and egg then mix well.
4. Take out the skillet and add the melted shortening into the batter and stir well.
5. Pour all mixed ingredients into the skillet.
6. For 15–20 minutes, cook in the oven until golden brown.

NUTRIENTS PER SERVING

- Calories: 166
- Protein 5 g.
- Carb: 35 g.
- Fat: 1 g.
- Sodium 34 mg.
- Potassium 122 mg.
- Phosphorus: 79mg.

5. Grandma's Pancake Special

PREPARATION TIME
5'

COOK TIME
15'

SERVING
3

INGREDIENTS

- 1 tbsp. oil
- 1 cup milk
- 1 egg
- 2 tsp. sodium-free baking powder
- 2 tbsp. sugar
- 1 1/4 cups flour

DIRECTIONS

1. Mix all the dry ingredients such as flour, sugar, and baking powder.
2. Combine oil, milk, and egg in another bowl. Once done, add them all to the flour mixture.
3. Make sure that as you stir the mixture, blend them until slightly lumpy.
4. In a hot greased griddle, pour-in at least 1/4 cup of the batter to make each pancake.
5. To cook, ensure that the bottom is a bit brown, then turn and cook the other side, as well.

NUTRIENTS PER SERVING

- Calories: 167
- Protein: 11 g.
- Carb: 50 g.
- Fats: 11 g.
- Sodium 70 mg.
- Potassium: 215 mg.
- Phosphorus: 176 mg.

6. Baked Egg Muffins

PREPARATION TIME
15'

COOK TIME
25'

SERVING
6

INGREDIENTS

- 1/3 cup onion, diced
- 1/3 cup mushrooms, diced
- 1/3 cup bell pepper, diced
- 1/2 cup turkey or chicken pieces, cooked, skinless
- 6 large eggs
- 1 tsp. dried thyme

DIRECTIONS

1. Line a muffin pan with 6 wrappers.
2. Mix vegetables in a separate bowl.
3. Next, spoon the vegetable mixture and turkey pieces into the muffin trays up to about 2-3 full, allowing room for the eggs.
4. Beat the eggs with the thyme in a separate bowl or jug.
5. Pour beaten eggs into each muffin tray—leave 1 cm. gap at the top.
6. Place the muffin tray in the oven and bake for approximately 25 minutes or until eggs are cooked through.
7. Remove egg muffins and serve.

NUTRIENTS PER SERVING

- Calories: 101
- Protein: 11 g.
- Fat: 5 g.
- Carb 3 g.
- Sodium: 222 mg.
- Potassium: 173 mg.
- Phosphorus: 141 mg.

7. Pasta With Indian Lentils

PREPARATION TIME

10’

COOK TIME

45’

SERVING

6

INGREDIENTS

- 1/4–1/2 cup fresh cilantro, chopped
- 3 cups of water
- 2 small dry red peppers, whole
- 1 tsp. turmeric
- 1 tsp. ground cumin
- 2?3 garlic cloves, minced
- 1 can (15 oz.) cubed tomatoes, with juice
- 1 large onion, chopped
- 1/2 cup dry lentils, rinsed
- 1 tbsp. vegetable oil
- 1/2 cup orzo or small pasta

DIRECTIONS

1. In a skillet, combine all ingredients except for the cilantro then boil on medium-high heat.
2. Ensure to cover and slightly reduce heat to medium-low and simmer for 25 minutes, add the pasta until pasta is tender for about 8 minutes.
3. Afterward, take out the chili peppers then add cilantro and top it with low-fat sour cream.

NUTRIENTS PER SERVING

- Calories: 170
- Carb: 29 g.
- Protein: 7 g.
- Fats: 3 g.
- Sodium: 168 mg.
- Potassium: 327 mg.
- Phosphorus: 139 mg.

8. Cherry-Pineapple Bread

PREPARATION TIME
20'

COOK TIME
1 HOUR

SERVING
10

INGREDIENTS

- 1/3 cup Swerve
- 1/3 cup butter, unsalted
- 2 eggs
- 2 cups flour
- 3 tsp. baking powder
- 1 cup pineapple, undrained
- 6 cherries, chopped
- 1/2 cup orzo or small pasta

DIRECTIONS

1. Whisk the Swerve with the butter in a mixer until fluffy.
2. Stir in the eggs, then beat again.
3. Add the baking powder and flour, then mix well until smooth.
4. Fold in the cherries and pineapple.
5. Spread this cherry-pineapple batter in a 9x5 inch baking pan.
6. Bake the pineapple batter for 1 hour at 350°F.
7. Slice the bread and serve.

NUTRIENTS PER SERVING

- Calories: 197
- Protein: 4 g.
- Fat: 7 g.
- Sodium: 85 mg.
- Potassium: 227 mg.
- Phosphorus: 316 mg.

9. Parmesan Zucchini Frittata

PREPARATION TIME
10'

COOK TIME
35'

SERVING
6

INGREDIENTS

- 1 tbsp. olive oil
- 1 cup yellow onion, sliced
- 3 cups zucchini, chopped
- 1/2 cup parmesan cheese, grated
- 8 large eggs
- 1/2 tsp. black pepper
- 1/8 tsp. paprika
- 3 tbsp. parsley, chopped

DIRECTIONS

1. Toss the zucchinis with the onion, parsley, and all other ingredients in a large bowl.
2. Pour this zucchini-garlic mixture into an 11x7 inches pan and spread it evenly.
3. Bake the zucchini casserole for approximately 35 minutes at 350°F.
4. Cut in slices and serve.

NUTRIENTS PER SERVING

- Calories: 142
- Protein: 10.2 g.
- Carb: 4.7 g.
- Fat: 9.7 g.
- Sodium: 123 mg.
- Potassium: 286 mg.
- Phosphorus: 375 mg.

10. Garlic Mayo Bread

PREPARATION TIME
10’

COOK TIME
5’

SERVING
16

INGREDIENTS

- 3 tbsp. vegetable oil
- 4 cloves garlic, minced
- 2 tsp. paprika
- Dash cayenne pepper
- 1 tsp. lemon juice
- 2 tbsp. parmesan cheese, grated
- 3/4 cup mayonnaise
- 1 loaf (1 lb.) French bread, sliced
- 1 tsp. Italian herbs

DIRECTIONS

1. Mix the garlic with the oil in a small bowl and leave it overnight.
2. Discard the garlic from the bowl and keep the garlic-infused oil.
3. Mix the garlic-oil with cayenne, paprika, lemon juice, mayonnaise, and parmesan.
4. Place the bread slices in a baking tray lined with parchment paper.
5. Top these slices with the mayonnaise mixture and drizzle the Italian herbs on top.
6. Broil these slices for 5 minutes until golden brown.
7. Serve warm.

NUTRIENTS PER SERVING

- Calories: 217
- Protein: 7 g.
- Fat: 7.9 g.
- Sodium: 423 mg.
- Potassium: 72 mg.
- Phosphorus: 347 mg.

11. Strawberry Topped Waffles

PREPARATION TIME
15'

COOK TIME
20'

SERVING
5

INGREDIENTS

- 1 cup flour
- 1/4 cup Swerve
- 1 3/4 tsp. baking powder
- 1 egg, separated
- 3/4 cup milk
- 1/2 cup butter, melted
- 1/2 tsp. vanilla extract
- Fresh strawberries, sliced

DIRECTIONS

1. Prepare and preheat your waffle pan following the instructions of the machine.
2. Begin by mixing the flour with Swerve and baking soda in a bowl.
3. Separate the egg yolks from the egg whites, keeping them in two separate bowls.
4. Add the milk and vanilla extract to the egg yolks.
5. Stir the melted butter and mix well until smooth.
6. Now beat the egg whites with an electric beater until foamy and fluffy.
7. Fold this fluffy composition in the egg yolk mixture.
8. Mix it gently until smooth, then add in the flour mixture.
9. Stir again to make a smooth mixture.
10. Pour a half cup of the waffle batter into a preheated pan and cook until the waffle is done.
11. Cook more waffles with the remaining batter.
12. Serve fresh with strawberries on top.

NUTRIENTS PER SERVING

- Calories: 342
- Protein: 4.8 g.
- Fat: 20.5 g.
- Sodium: 156 mg.
- Potassium: 233 mg.
- Phosphorus: 126 mg.

12. Cheese Spaghetti Frittata

PREPARATION TIME
10’

COOK TIME
10’

SERVING
6

INGREDIENTS

- 4 cups whole-wheat spaghetti, cooked
- 4 tsp. olive oil
- 3 medium onions, chopped
- 4 large eggs
- 1/2 cup milk
- 1/3 cup parmesan cheese, grated
- 2 tbsp. fresh parsley, chopped
- 2 tbsp. fresh basil, chopped
- 1/2 tsp. black pepper
- 1 tomato, diced

DIRECTIONS

1. Set a suitable non-stick skillet over moderate heat and add in the olive oil.
2. Place the spaghetti in the skillet and cook by stirring for 2 minutes on moderate heat.
3. Whisk the eggs with milk, parsley, and black pepper in a bowl.
4. Pour this milky egg mixture over the spaghetti and top it all with basil, cheese, and tomato.
5. Cover the spaghetti frittata again with a lid and cook for approximately 8 minutes on low heat.
6. Slice and serve.

NUTRIENTS PER SERVING

- Calories: 230
- Protein: 11 g.
- Fat: 7.8 g.
- Sodium: 77 mg.
- Potassium: 214 mg.
- Phosphorus: 368 mg.

13. Shrimp Bruschetta

PREPARATION TIME
15'

COOK TIME
10'

SERVING
4

INGREDIENTS

- 13 oz. shrimps, peeled
- 1 tbsp. tomato sauce
- 1/2 tsp. Splenda
- 1/4 tsp. garlic powder
- 1 tsp. fresh parsley, chopped
- 1/2 tsp. olive oil
- 1 tsp. lemon juice
- 4 whole-grain bread slices
- 1 cup water, for cooking

DIRECTIONS

1. In the saucepan, pour water and bring it to a boil.
2. Add shrimps and boil them over the high heat for 5 minutes.
3. After this, drain shrimps and chill them to room temperature.
4. Mix up together shrimps with Splenda, garlic powder, tomato sauce, and fresh parsley.
5. Add lemon juice and stir gently.
6. Preheat the oven to 360°F.
7. Coat the slice of bread with olive oil and bake for 3 minutes.
8. Then place the shrimp mixture on the bread. Bruschetta is cooked.

NUTRIENTS PER SERVING

- Calories: 199
- Protein: 24 g.
- Carb: 15.3 g.
- Fat: 3.7 g.
- Sodium: 121 mg.
- Potassium: 227 mg.
- Phosphorus: 316 mg.

14. Strawberry & Blueberry Muesli

PREPARATION TIME
10'

COOK TIME
30'

SERVING
4

INGREDIENTS

- 2 cups Greek yogurt
- 1 1/2 cup strawberries, sliced
- 1 1/2 cup blueberries, sliced
- 1 1/2 cup muesli
- 4 tsp. maple syrup
- 3/4 tsp. ground cinnamon

DIRECTIONS

1. Put Greek yogurt in the food processor.
2. Add 1 cup of strawberries, maple syrup, and ground cinnamon.
3. Blend the ingredients until you get smooth mass.
4. Transfer the yogurt mass to the serving bowls.
5. Add the muesli and stir well.
6. Leave the meal for 30 minutes in the fridge.
7. After this, decorate it with the remaining sliced strawberries.

NUTRIENTS PER SERVING

- Calories: 149
- Protein: 12 g.
- Fat: 2.6 g.
- Carb: 21.6 g.
- Sodium: 151 mg.
- Potassium: 227 mg.
- Phosphorus: 216 mg.

15. Mexican Style Burritos

PREPARATION TIME
5'

COOK TIME
15'

SERVING
2

INGREDIENTS

- 2 white tortillas
- 1 tbsp. canola oil
- 1/4 cup red onion, diced
- 1/2 red chili, de-seeded and finely chopped
- 1/4 cup red bell peppers, diced
- 2 eggs
- 1 tbsp. cilantro, finely chopped
- 1 lime, freshly squeezed

DIRECTIONS

1. Turn the broiler to medium heat and place the tortillas underneath for 1–2 minutes on each side or until lightly toasted. Place to one side but keep broiler on.
2. Now heat the oil in a skillet over medium heat and sauté the onion, chili, and bell peppers for 5–6 minutes until soft.
3. Crack the eggs over the top of the onions and peppers and place the skillet under the broiler for 5–6 minutes or until the eggs are cooked.
4. Serve half the eggs and vegetables on top of each tortilla and sprinkle with cilantro and lime juice to serve.

NUTRIENTS PER SERVING

- Calories: 197
- Protein: 7 g.
- Fat: 12 g.
- Carb: 17 g.
- Sodium: 201 mg.
- Potassium: 208 mg.
- Phosphorus: 178 mg.

CHAPTER 12

Alternative Yummy Main Dishes

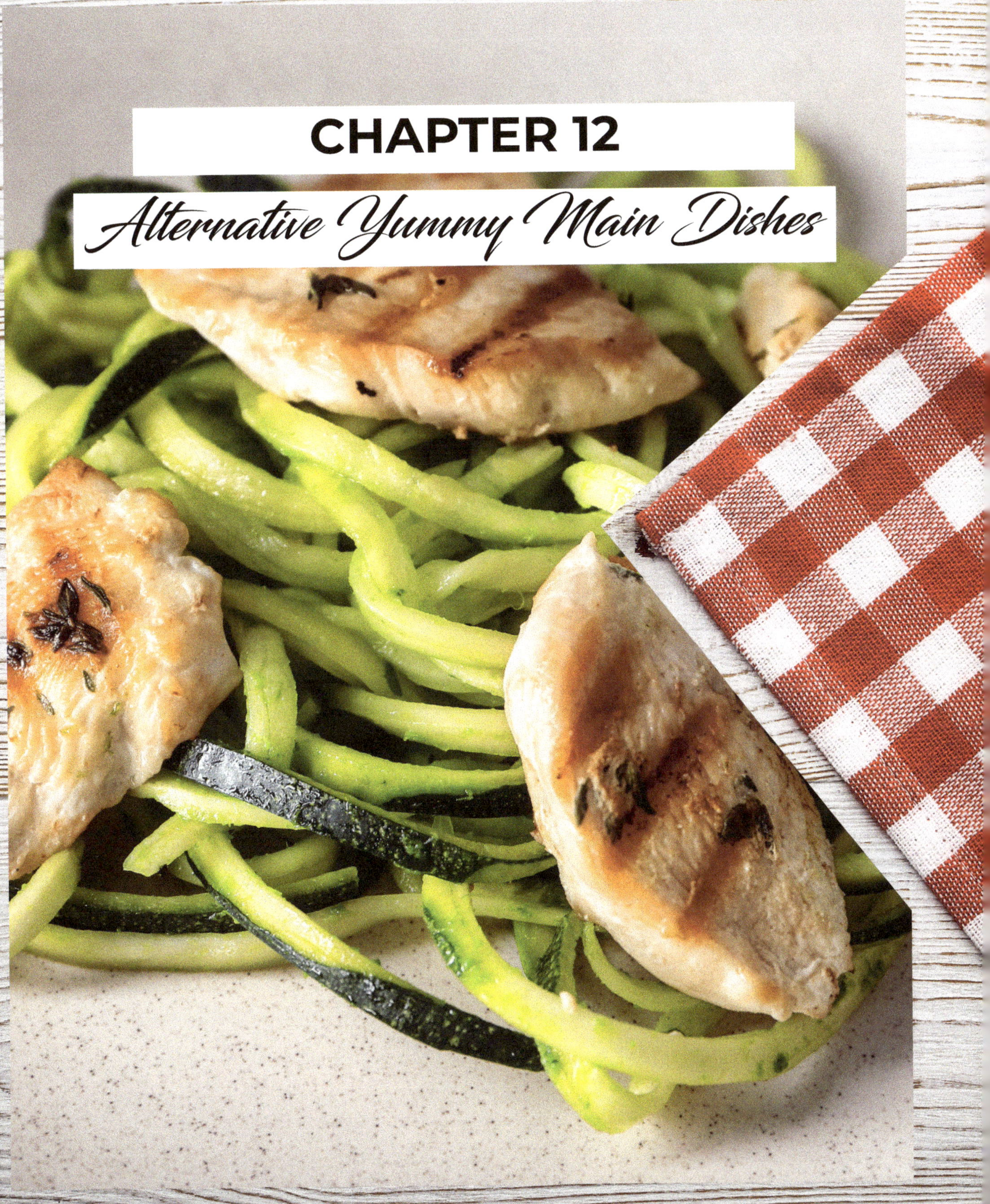

16. Light Paprika Moussaka

PREPARATION TIME
15'

COOK TIME
45'

SERVING
3

INGREDIENTS

- 1 eggplant, trimmed
- 1 cup ground chicken
- 1/3 cup white onion, diced
- 3 oz. cheddar cheese, shredded
- 1 potato, sliced
- 1 tsp. olive oil
- 1 tsp. salt
- 1/2 cup milk
- 1 tbsp. butter
- 1 tbsp. ground paprika
- 1 tbsp. Italian seasoning
- 1 tsp. tomato paste

DIRECTIONS

1. Slice the eggplant lengthwise and sprinkle with salt.
2. Pour olive oil into the skillet and add sliced potato.
3. Roast potato for 2 minutes from each side.
4. Then transfer it to the plate.
5. Put eggplant in the skillet and roast it for 2 minutes from each side too.
6. Pour milk into the pan and bring it to a boil.
7. Add tomato paste, Italian seasoning, paprika, butter, and cheddar cheese.
8. Then mix up together onion with ground chicken.
9. Arrange the sliced potato in the casserole in one layer.
10. Then add 1/2 part of all sliced eggplants.
11. Spread the eggplants with 1/2 part of the chicken mixture.
12. Then add the remaining eggplants.
13. Pour the milk mixture over the eggplants.
14. Bake moussaka for 30 minutes at 355°F.

NUTRIENTS PER SERVING

- Calories: 387
- Protein: 25.4 g.
- Fat: 21.2 g.
- Carb: 26.3 g.
- Sodium: 121 mg.
- Potassium: 227 mg.
- Phosphorus: 316 mg.

17. Cucumber Bowl With Spices and Greek Yogurt

PREPARATION TIME
10'

COOK TIME
20'

SERVING
3

INGREDIENTS

- 4 cucumbers
- 1/2 tsp. chili pepper
- 1/4 cup fresh parsley, chopped
- 3/4 cup fresh dill, chopped
- 2 tbsp. lemon juice
- 1/2 tsp. salt
- 1/2 tsp. ground black pepper
- 1/4 tsp. sage
- 1/2 tsp. dried oregano
- 1/3 cup Greek yogurt

DIRECTIONS

1. Make the cucumber dressing: blend the dill and parsley until you get green mash.
2. Then combine green mash with lemon juice, salt, ground black pepper, sage, dried oregano, Greek yogurt, and chili pepper.
3. Churn the mixture well.
4. Chop the cucumbers roughly and combine them with cucumber dressing. Mix up well.
5. Refrigerate the cucumber for 20 minutes.

NUTRIENTS PER SERVING

- Calories: 114
- Protein: 7.6 g.
- Fat: 1.6 g.
- Carb: 23.2 g.
- Sodium: 181 mg.
- Potassium: 217 mg.
- Phosphorus: 250 mg.

18. Stuffed Bell Peppers With Quinoa

PREPARATION TIME
15'

COOK TIME
35'

SERVING
2

INGREDIENTS

- 2 bell peppers
- 1/3 cup quinoa
- 3 oz. chicken stock
- 1/4 cup onion, diced
- 1/2 tsp. salt
- 1/4 tsp. tomato paste
- 1/2 tsp. dried oregano
- 1/3 cup sour cream
- 1 tsp. paprika

DIRECTIONS

1. Trim the bell peppers and remove the seeds.
2. Then combine chicken stock and quinoa in the pan.
3. Add salt and boil the ingredients for 10 minutes or until quinoa will soak all liquid.
4. Then combine cooked quinoa with dried oregano, tomato paste, and onion.
5. Fill the bell peppers with the quinoa mixture and arrange in the casserole mold.
6. Add sour cream and bake the peppers for 25 minutes at 365°F.
7. Serve the cooked peppers with sour cream sauce from the casserole mold.

NUTRIENTS PER SERVING

- Calories: 237
- Protein: 6.9 g.
- Fat: 10.3 g.
- Carb: 31.3 g.
- Sodium: 121 mg.
- Potassium: 227 mg.
- Phosphorus: 316 mg.

19. Mediterranean Burrito

PREPARATION TIME
10'

COOK TIME
0'

SERVING
2

INGREDIENTS

- 2 wheat tortillas
- 2 oz. red kidney beans, canned, drained
- 2 tbsp. hummus
- 2 tsp. tahini sauce
- 1 cucumber
- 2 lettuce leaves
- 1 tbsp. lime juice
- 1 tsp. olive oil
- 1/2 tsp. dried oregano

DIRECTIONS

1. Mash the red kidney beans until you get a puree.
2. Then spread the wheat tortillas with beans mash from one side.
3. Add hummus and tahini sauce.
4. Cut the cucumber into the wedges and place them over tahini sauce.
5. Then add lettuce leaves.
6. Make the dressing: mix up together olive oil, dried oregano, and lime juice.
7. Drizzle the lettuce leaves with the dressing and wrap the wheat tortillas in the shape of burritos.

NUTRIENTS PER SERVING

- Calories: 288
- Protein: 12.5 g.
- Fat: 10.2 g.
- Carb: 38.2 g.
- Sodium: 191 mg.
- Potassium: 207 mg.
- Phosphorus: 216 mg.

20. Sweet Potato Bacon Mash

PREPARATION TIME
10'

COOK TIME
20'

SERVING
4

INGREDIENTS

- 3 sweet potatoes, peeled
- 4 oz. bacon, chopped
- 1 cup chicken stock
- 1 tbsp. butter
- 1 tsp. salt
- 2 oz. parmesan, grated

DIRECTIONS

1. Chop sweet potato and put it in the pan.
2. Add chicken stock and close the lid.
3. Boil the vegetables for 15 minutes or until they are soft.
4. After this, drain the chicken stock.
5. Mash the sweet potato with the help of the potato masher. Add grated cheese and butter.
6. Mix up together salt and chopped bacon. Fry the mixture until it is crunchy (10–15 minutes).
7. Add cooked bacon to the mashed sweet potato and mix up with the help of the spoon.
8. It is recommended to serve the meal warm or hot.

NUTRIENTS PER SERVING

- Calories: 304
- Protein: 17 g.
- Fat: 18.1 g.
- Carb: 18.8 g.
- Sodium: 121 mg.
- Potassium: 227 mg.
- Phosphorus 316 mg.

21. Prosciutto Wrapped Mozzarella Balls

PREPARATION TIME

10'

COOK TIME

10'

SERVING

4

INGREDIENTS

- 8 mozzarella balls, cherry size
- 4 oz. bacon, sliced
- 1/4 tsp. ground black pepper
- 3/4 tsp. dried rosemary
- 1 tsp. butter

DIRECTIONS

1. Sprinkle the sliced bacon with ground black pepper and dried rosemary.
2. Wrap every mozzarella ball in the sliced bacon and secure them with toothpicks.
3. Melt butter.
4. Brush wrapped mozzarella balls with butter.
5. Line the tray with the baking paper and arrange mozzarella balls in it.
6. Bake the meal for 10 minutes at 365°F.

NUTRIENTS PER SERVING

- Calories: 323
- Protein: 20.6 g.
- Fat: 26.8 g.
- Carb: 0.6 g.
- Sodium: 181 mg.
- Potassium: 237 mg.
- Phosphorus: 296 mg.

22. Garlic Chicken Balls

PREPARATION TIME
15'

COOK TIME
10'

SERVING
4

INGREDIENTS

- 2 cups ground chicken
- 1 tsp. garlic, minced
- 1 tsp. dried dill
- 1/3 carrot, grated
- 1 egg, beaten
- 1 tbsp. olive oil
- 1/4 cup coconut flakes
- 1/2 tsp. salt

DIRECTIONS

1. In the mixing bowl mix up together ground chicken, minced garlic, dried dill, carrot, egg, and salt.
2. Stir the chicken mixture with the help of the fingertips until homogenous.
3. Then make medium balls from the mixture.
4. Coat every chicken ball in coconut flakes.
5. Heat olive oil in the skillet.
6. Add chicken balls and cook them for 3 minutes from each side. The cooked chicken balls will have a golden-brown color.

NUTRIENTS PER SERVING

- Calories: 200
- Protein: 21.9 g.
- Fat: 11.5 g.
- Carb: 1.7 g.
- Sodium: 161 mg.
- Potassium: 217 mg.
- Phosphorus: 216 mg.

23. Jarlsberg Omelet

PREPARATION TIME
5'

COOK TIME
10'

SERVING
2

INGREDIENTS

- 4 medium mushrooms, sliced, 2 oz.
- 1 green onion, sliced
- 2 eggs, beaten
- 1 oz. Jarlsberg or Swiss cheese, shredded
- 1 oz. ham, diced

DIRECTIONS

1. In a skillet, cook the mushrooms and green onion until tender.
2. Add the eggs and mix well.
3. Sprinkle with salt and top with the mushroom mixture, cheese, and ham.
4. When the egg is set, fold the plain side of the omelet on the filled side.
5. Turn off the heat and let it stand until the cheese has melted.
6. Serve!

NUTRIENTS PER SERVING

- Calories: 288
- Protein: 27 g.
- Fat: 12 g.
- Carb: 22 g.
- Sodium: 121 mg.
- Potassium: 227 mg.
- Phosphorus: 316 mg.

24. Mu Shu Pork

PREPARATION TIME
5'

COOK TIME
10'

SERVING
2

INGREDIENTS

- 4 cups coleslaw mix, with carrots
- 1 small onion, sliced thin
- 1 lb. cooked roast pork, cut into 1/2" cubes
- 2 tbsp. hoisin sauce
- 2 tbsp. soy sauce

DIRECTIONS

1. In a large skillet, heat the oil on high heat.
2. Stir-fry the cabbage and onion for 4 minutes until tender.
3. Add the pork, hoisin, and soy sauce.
4. Cook until browned.
5. Enjoy!

NUTRIENTS PER SERVING

- Calories: 388
- Protein: 25 g.
- Fat: 21 g.
- Carb: 16 g.
- Sodium: 121 mg.
- Potassium: 127 mg.
- Phosphorus: 287 mg.

25. Fiery Jalapeño Poppers

PREPARATION TIME
10'

COOK TIME
40'

SERVING
4

INGREDIENTS

- 5 oz. cream cheese
- 1/4 cup mozzarella cheese
- 8 medium jalapeño peppers
- 1/2 tsp. Mrs. Dash Table Blend®
- 8 slices bacon

DIRECTIONS

1. Preheat your fryer to 400°F (200°C).
2. Cut the jalapeños in half.
3. Use a spoon to scrape out the insides of the peppers.
4. In a bowl, add together the cream cheese, mozzarella cheese, and spices of your choice.
5. Pack the cream cheese mixture into the jalapeños and place the peppers on top.
6. Wrap each pepper in 1 slice of bacon, starting from the bottom and working up.
7. Bake for 30 minutes. Broil for an additional 3 minutes.
8. Serve!

NUTRIENTS PER SERVING

- Calories: 238
- Protein: 24 g.
- Fat: 10 g.
- Carb: 4 g.
- Sodium: 145 mg.
- Potassium: 228 mg.
- Phosphorus: 316 mg.

26. Bacon & Chicken Patties

PREPARATION TIME
5'

COOK TIME
15'

SERVING
2

INGREDIENTS

- 1 1/2 oz. can chicken breast
- 4 slices bacon
- 1/4 cup parmesan cheese
- 1 large egg
- 3 tbsp. flour

DIRECTIONS

1. Cook the bacon until crispy.
2. Chop the chicken and bacon together in a food processor until fine.
3. Add in the parmesan, egg, flour, and mix.
4. Make the patties by hand and fry on medium heat in a pan with some oil.
5. Once browned, flip over, continue cooking, and lie them to drain.
6. Serve!

NUTRIENTS PER SERVING

- Calories: 387
- Protein: 34 g.
- Fat: 16 g.
- Carb: 13 g.
- Sodium: 121 mg.
- Potassium: 197 mg.
- Phosphorus: 226 mg.

27. Cheddar Bacon Burst

PREPARATION TIME

25'

COOK TIME

90'

SERVING

8

INGREDIENTS

- 30 slices bacon
- 2 1/2 cups cheddar cheese
- 4–5 cups raw spinach
- 1–2 tbsp. Tones Southwest Chipotle Seasoning
- 2 tsp. Mrs. Dash Table Seasoning (dash salt-free seasoning blend)

DIRECTIONS

1. Preheat your fryer to 375°F/190°C.
2. Weave the bacon into 15 vertical pieces and 12 horizontal pieces. Cut the extra 3 in half to fill in the rest, horizontally.
3. Season the bacon.
4. Add the cheese to the bacon.
5. Add the spinach and press down to compress.
6. Tightly roll up the woven bacon.
7. Line a baking sheet with kitchen foil and add plenty of salt to it.
8. Put the bacon on top of a cooling rack and put that on top of your baking sheet.
9. Bake for 60–70 minutes.
10. Let cool for 10–15 minutes before
11. Slice and enjoy!

NUTRIENTS PER SERVING

- Calories: 259
- Protein: 16 g.
- Fat: 20 g.
- Carb: 2 g.
- Sodium: 161 mg.
- Potassium: 227 mg.
- Phosphorus: 236 mg.

28. Grilled Ham & Cheese

PREPARATION TIME
15'

COOK TIME
30'

SERVING
2

INGREDIENTS

- 4 slices medium-cut deli ham
- 2 low-carb buns
- 1 tbsp. butter
- 1 oz. coconut flour
- 2 slices cheddar cheese
- 2 slices muenster cheese
- 2 eggs
- Coconut oil

DIRECTIONS

1. **Bread:**
2. Preheat your fryer to 350°F/175°C.
3. Mix the flour, salt, and baking powder in a bowl. Put to the side.
4. Add the butter and coconut oil to a skillet.
5. Melt for 20 seconds and pour into another bowl.
6. In this bowl, mix in the dough.
7. Scramble 2 eggs. Add to the dough.
8. Add 1/2 tbsp. of coconut flour to thicken, and place evenly into a cupcake tray. Fill about 3/4 inch.
9. Bake for 20 minutes until browned.
10. Allow to cool for 15 minutes and cut each in half for the buns.
11. **Sandwich:**
12. Fry the deli meat in a skillet on high heat.
13. Put the ham and cheese between the buns.
14. Heat the butter on medium-high.
15. When brown, turn to low and add the dough to the pan.
16. Press down with weight until you smell burning, then flip to crisp both sides.
17. Enjoy!

NUTRIENTS PER SERVING

- Calories: 200
- Protein: 14 g.
- Fat: 16 g.
- Carb: 12 g.
- Sodium: 121 mg.
- Potassium: 227 mg.
- Phosphorus 316 mg.

29. Mashed Garlic Turnips

PREPARATION TIME
5'

COOK TIME
10'

SERVING
2

INGREDIENTS

- 3 cups diced turnip
- 2 cloves garlic, minced
- 1/4 cup heavy cream
- 3 tbsp. melted butter
- Salt and pepper to season

DIRECTIONS

1. Boil the turnips until tender.
2. Drain and mash the turnips.
3. Add the cream, butter, salt, pepper, and garlic. Combine well.
4. Serve!

NUTRIENTS PER SERVING

- Calories: 488
- Protein: 34 g.
- Fat: 19 g.
- Carb: 32 g.
- Sodium: 189 mg.
- Potassium: 218 mg.
- Phosphorus: 266 mg.

30. Lasagna Spaghetti Squash

PREPARATION TIME
30'

COOK TIME
90'

SERVING
6

INGREDIENTS

- 2 large spaghetti squash, cooked (44 oz.)
- 4 lb. ground beef
- 25 slices mozzarella cheese
- 1 large jar (40 oz.) Rao's Marinara sauce (Italian-style sauce: tomatoes, basil, olive oil, minced onions, peeled minced garlic, oregano, salt, and pepper)
- 30 oz. whole-milk ricotta cheese

DIRECTIONS

1. Preheat your fryer to 375°F/190°C.
2. Slice the spaghetti squash and place it face down inside a fryer proof dish. Fill with water until covered.
3. Bake for 45 minutes until the skin is soft.
4. Sear the meat until browned.
5. In a large skillet, heat the browned meat and marinara sauce. Set aside when warm.
6. Scrape the flesh off the cooked squash to resemble strands of spaghetti.
7. Layer the lasagna in a large greased pan in alternating layers of spaghetti squash, meat sauce, mozzarella, ricotta. Repeat until all have been used.
8. Bake for 30 minutes and serve!

NUTRIENTS PER SERVING

- Calories: 508
- Protein: 22 g.
- Fat: 8 g.
- Carb: 32 g.
- Sodium: 121 mg.
- Potassium: 245 mg.
- Phosphorus: 312 mg.

CHAPTER 13

Fish and Seafood

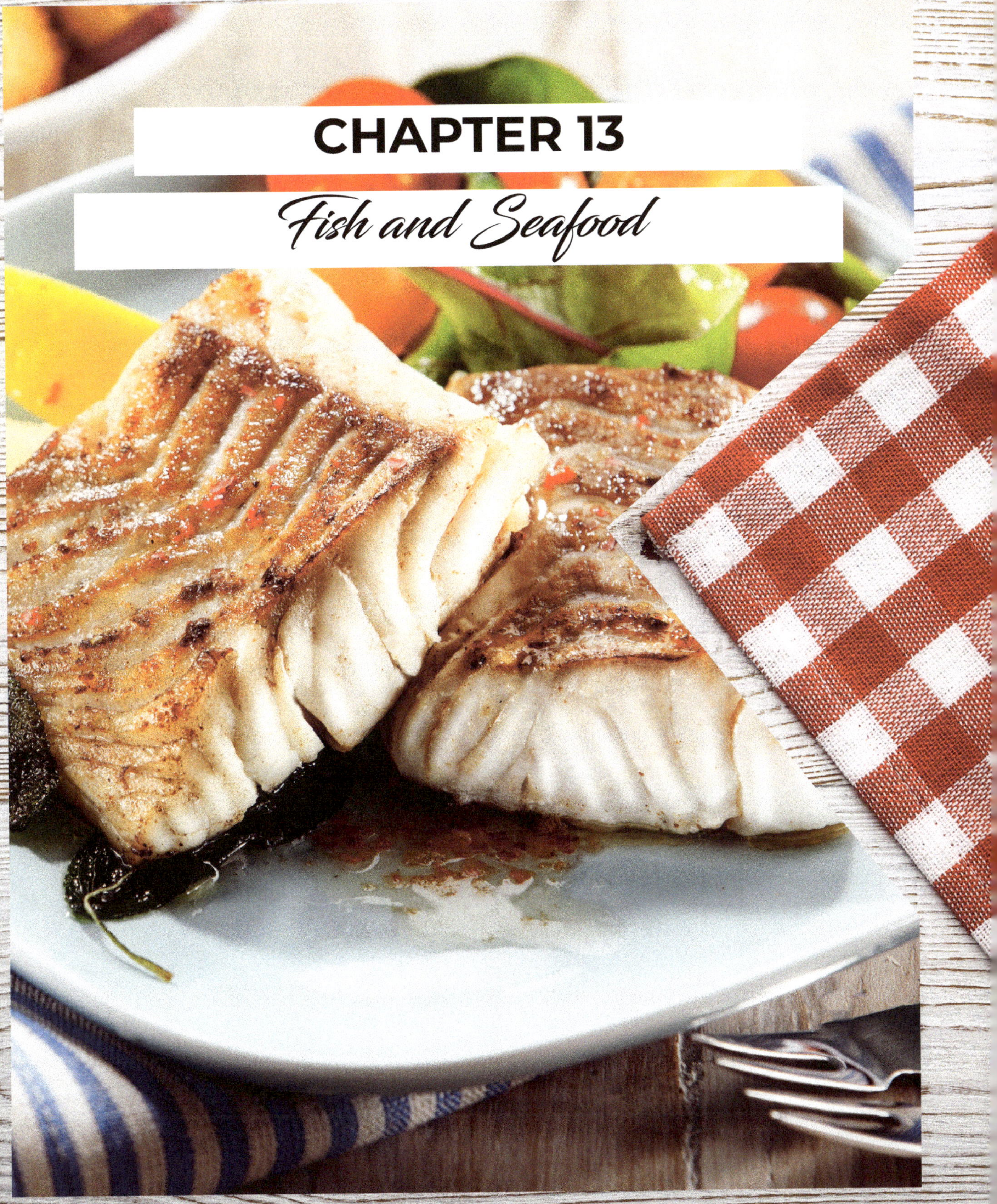

31. Salmon Stuffed Pasta Shells

PREPARATION TIME

20'

COOK TIME

35'

SERVING

6 (1 SERVING = 4 SHELLS)

INGREDIENTS

- 24 jumbo pasta shells, boiled
- 1 cup coffee creamer

Filling:

- 2 eggs, beaten
- 2 cups creamed cottage cheese
- 1/4 cup onion, chopped
- 1 red bell pepper, diced
- 2 tsp. dried parsley t
- 1/2 tsp. lemon peel
- 1 can salmon, drained

Dill Sauce:

- 1 1/2 tsp. butter
- 1 1/2 tsp. flour
- 1/8 tsp. pepper
- 1 tbsp. lemon juice
- 1 1/2 cup coffee creamer
- 2 tsp. dried dill weed

DIRECTIONS

1. Cook pasta and drain
2. Whip the egg with the cream cheese and all the other filling ingredients in a bowl.
3. Divide the filling in the pasta shells and place the shells in a 9x13 baking dish.
4. Pour the coffee creamer around the stuffed shells then cover with a foil.
5. Bake the shells for 30 minutes at 350°F.
6. Meanwhile, whisk all the ingredients for dill sauce in a saucepan.
7. Stir for 5 minutes until it thickens.
8. Pour this sauce over the baked pasta shells.
9. Serve warm.

NUTRIENTS PER SERVING

- Calories 370
- Protein: 24 g.
- Fat: 12 g.
- Carb: 40 g.
- Sodium: 86 mg.
- Potassium: 181 mg.
- Phosphorus: 314 mg.

32. Herbed Vegetable Trout

PREPARATION TIME
15'

COOK TIME
15'

SERVING
4

INGREDIENTS

- 14 oz. trout fillets
- 1/2 tsp. herb seasoning blend
- 1 lemon, sliced
- 2 green onions, sliced
- 1 stalk celery, chopped
- 1 medium carrot, julienne

Dill Sauce:

- 1 1/2 tsp. butter
- 1 1/2 tsp. flour
- 1/8 tsp. pepper
- 1 tbsp. lemon juice
- 1 1/2 cup coffee creamer
- 2 tsp. dried dill weed

DIRECTIONS

1. Prepare and preheat a charcoal grill over moderate heat.
2. Place the trout fillets over a large piece of foil and drizzle herb seasoning on top.
3. Spread the lemon slices, carrots, celery, and green onions over the fish.
4. Cover the fish with foil and pack it.
5. Place the packed fish in the grill and cook for 15 minutes.
6. Once done, remove the foil from the fish.

NUTRIENTS PER SERVING

- Calories 202
- Protein: 21 g.
- Fat 7 g.
- Carb: 4 g.
- Sodium: 59 mg.
- Potassium: 529 mg.
- Phosphorus: 249 mg.

33. Citrus Glazed Salmon

PREPARATION TIME
20'

COOK TIME
17'

SERVING
6

INGREDIENTS

- 24 oz. salmon filet
- 2 garlic cloves, crushed
- 1 1/2 tbsp. lemon juice
- 2 tbsp. olive oil
- 1 tbsp. butter
- 1 tbsp. Dijon mustard
- 2 dashes cayenne pepper
- 1 tsp. dried basil leaves
- 1 tsp. dried dill

DIRECTIONS

1. Place 1-quart saucepan over moderate heat and add the oil, butter, garlic, lemon juice, mustard, cayenne pepper, dill, and basil to the pan.
2. Stir this mixture for 5 minutes after it has boiled.
3. Prepare and preheat a charcoal grill over moderate heat.
4. Place the fish on a foil sheet and fold the edges to make a foil tray.
5. Pour the prepared sauce over the fish.
6. Place the fish in the foil in the preheated grill and cook for 12 minutes.

NUTRIENTS PER SERVING

- Calories 401
- Protein: 24 g.
- Fat: 21 g.
- Carb: 1 g.
- Sodium: 199 mg.
- Potassium: 429 mg.
- Phosphorus: 279 mg.

34. Broiled Salmon Fillets

PREPARATION TIME
10'

COOK TIME
13'

SERVING
4

INGREDIENTS

- 4 salmon fillets, skinless
- 1 tbsp. ginger root, grated
- 1 clove garlic, minced
- 1/4 cup maple syrup
- 1 tbsp. hot pepper sauce

DIRECTIONS

1. Grease a pan with cooking spray and place it over moderate heat.
2. Add the ginger and garlic and sauté for 3 minutes then transfer to a bowl.
3. Add the hot pepper sauce and maple syrup to the ginger-garlic.
4. Mix well and keep this mixture aside.
5. Place the salmon fillet in a suitable baking tray, greased with cooking oil.
6. Brush the maple sauce over the fillets liberally.
7. Broil them for 10 minutes in the oven at broiler settings.
8. Serve warm.

NUTRIENTS PER SERVING

- Calories: 289
- Protein: 19 g.
- Fat: 14 g.
- Carb: 12 g.
- Sodium: 80 mg.
- Potassium: 331 mg.
- Phosphorus: 230 mg.

35. Broiled Shrimp

PREPARATION TIME
10'

COOK TIME
5'

SERVING
8

INGREDIENTS

- 1 lb. shrimp in shell
- 1/2 cup unsalted butter, melted
- 2 tsp. lemon juice
- 2 tbsp. onion, chopped
- 1 clove garlic, minced
- 1/8 tsp. pepper

DIRECTIONS

1. Toss the shrimp with the butter, lemon juice, onion, garlic, and pepper in a bowl.
2. Spread the seasoned shrimp in a baking tray.
3. Broil for 5 minutes in an oven on broiler setting.
4. Serve warm.

NUTRIENTS PER SERVING

- Calories 164
- Protein: 15 g.
- Fat 12.8 g.
- Carb: 0.6 g.
- Sodium: 242 mg.
- Potassium: 228 mg.
- Phosphorus 215 mg.

36. Grilled Lemony Cod

PREPARATION TIME

31

COOK TIME

10'

SERVING

4

INGREDIENTS

- 1 lb. cod fillets
- 1 tsp. salt-free lemon pepper seasoning
- 1/4 cup lemon juice

DIRECTIONS

1. Rub the cod fillets with lemon pepper seasoning and lemon juice.
2. Grease a baking tray with cooking spray and place the salmon in the baking tray.
3. Bake the fish for 10 minutes at 350°F in a preheated oven.
4. Serve warm.

NUTRIENTS PER SERVING

- Calories: 155
- Protein: 22 g.
- Fat: 7.1 g.
- Sodium: 53 mg.
- Potassium: 461 mg.
- Phosphorus: 237 mg.

37. Spiced Honey Salmon

PREPARATION TIME
15'

COOK TIME
16'

SERVING
4

INGREDIENTS

- 16 oz. salmon fillets
- 3 tbsp. honey
- 3/4 tsp. lemon peel
- 1/2 tsp. black pepper
- 1/2 tsp. garlic powder
- 1 tsp. water
- 2 tbsp. olive oil
- Dill, chopped, to serve

DIRECTIONS

1. Whisk the lemon peel with honey, garlic powder, hot water, and ground pepper in a small bowl.
2. Rub this honey mixture over the salmon fillet liberally.
3. Set a suitable skillet over moderate heat and add olive oil to heat.
4. Set the spiced salmon fillets in the pan and sear them for 4 minutes per side.
5. Garnish with dill.
6. Serve warm.

NUTRIENTS PER SERVING

- Calories: 264
- Protein: 24 g.
- Fat: 19 g.
- Carb: 14 g.
- Sodium: 59 mg.
- Potassium: 450 mg.
- Phosphorus: 259 mg.

38. Thai Fish Soup

PREPARATION TIME
25'

COOK TIME
20'

SERVING
4

INGREDIENTS

- 4 white fish fillets (medium size)
- 1/2 cup long-grain rice
- 1 clove chopped garlic
- 1/2 cup chopped green onion
- 1 cup celery, diced
- 1/2 tbsp. ginger, minced
- Basil
- Cilantro
- Mint
- Black pepper
- Lime
- 3 cups of boiling water

DIRECTIONS

1. Sauté ginger, garlic, celery, and green onion in 1 tbsp. oil.
2. Add water, fish, and celery.
3. Simmer until fish is cooked. Add herbs and black pepper.
4. Add cooked rice and serve warm.
5. Add herbs and a squeeze of lime juice.
6. Add dried chilies if you prefer it spicy.

NUTRIENTS PER SERVING

- Calories 80
- Protein: 4 g.
- Fat: 1.8 g.
- Carb: 10 g.
- Sodium: 75 mg.
- Potassium 180 mg.
- Phosphorus 49 mg.

39. Seared Herbed Scallops

PREPARATION TIME
10'

COOK TIME
15'

SERVING
4 (SERVING SIZE: 3 SCALLOPS)

INGREDIENTS

- 12 oz. sea scallops
- 1 tbsp. olive oil
- 1 tbsp. parsley, chopped
- 1 tbsp. thyme, chopped
- 1 tbsp. lemon juice
- 1 tbsp. chives, chopped
- Black pepper

DIRECTIONS

1. In a skillet heat oil, add scallops seasoned with pepper, and sear until scallops are cooked (about 5 minutes)
2. Stir in the lemon juice and herbs, turn the scallops in this sauce, and serve warm.

NUTRIENTS PER SERVING

- Calories: 121
- Protein: 13 g.
- Fat: 5 g.
- Carb: 3 g.
- Sodium: 269 mg.
- Potassium: 199 mg.
- Phosphorus: 239 mg.

40. Miso-Glazed Salmon

PREPARATION TIME
10'

COOK TIME
40'

SERVING
4

INGREDIENTS

- 4 salmon fillets
- 1/4 cup red miso
- 1/4 cup sake
- 1 tbsp. soy sauce
- 1 tbsp. vegetable oil

DIRECTIONS

1. In a bowl combine sake, oil, soy sauce, and miso.
2. Rub mixture over salmon fillets and marinate for 20⍰30 minutes.
3. Preheat a broiler.
4. Broil salmon for 5⍰10 minutes.
5. When ready, remove and serve.

NUTRIENTS PER SERVING

- Calories: 219
- Protein: 22 g.
- Fat: 10 g.
- Carb: 5 g.
- Sodium: 257 mg.
- Potassium: 222 mg.
- Phosphorus: 267 mg.

41. Fish Packets

PREPARATION TIME
15’

COOK TIME
20’

SERVING
3

INGREDIENTS

- 3 tilapia fillets (4 oz. each fish fillet)
- 1/2 tsp. cayenne pepper
- 1/2 tsp. salt
- 3 tsp. olive oil
- 1 red onion, sliced
- 3 lemon slices
- 1 zucchini, chopped

DIRECTIONS

1. Make the medium packets from the foil and brush them with olive oil from inside.
2. Then sprinkle tilapia fillets with salt and cayenne pepper from each side and arrange in the foil packets.
3. Add sliced lemon to the top of the fish.
4. Then add sliced onion and zucchini.
5. Bake the fish packets for 20 minutes at 360°F or until vegetables are tender.

NUTRIENTS PER SERVING

- Calories: 161
- Protein: 22.3 g.
- Fat: 5.9 g.
- Carb: 6.4 g.
- Sodium: 151 mg.
- Potassium: 257 mg.
- Phosphorus: 216 mg.

42. Salmon Baked in Foil With Fresh Thyme

PREPARATION TIME
10’

COOK TIME
30’

SERVING
4

INGREDIENTS

- 4 fresh thyme sprig
- 4 garlic cloves, peeled, roughly chopped
- 16 oz. salmon fillets (4 oz. each fillet)
- 1/2 tsp. salt
- 1/2 tsp. ground black pepper
- 4 tbsp. cream
- 4 tsp. butter
- 1/4 tsp. cumin seeds

DIRECTIONS

1. Line the baking tray with foil.
2. Sprinkle the fish fillets with salt, ground black pepper, cumin seeds, and arrange them in the tray with oil.
3. Add thyme sprig on the top of every fillet.
4. Then add cream, butter, and garlic.
5. Bake the fish for 30 minutes at 345°F.

NUTRIENTS PER SERVING

- Calories: 198
- Protein: 22.4 g.
- Fat: 11.6 g.
- Carb: 1.8 g.
- Sodium: 121 mg.
- Potassium: 245 mg.
- Phosphorus: 216 mg.

43. Poached Halibut in Orange Sauce

PREPARATION TIME

10’

COOK TIME

10’

SERVING

4

INGREDIENTS

- 1 lb. halibut
- 1/3 cup butter
- 1 rosemary sprig
- 1/2 tsp. ground black pepper
- 1 tsp. salt
- 1 tsp. honey
- 1/4 cup of orange juice
- 1 tsp. cornstarch

DIRECTIONS

1. Put butter in the saucepan and melt it.
2. Add rosemary sprig.
3. Sprinkle the halibut with salt and ground black pepper.
4. Put the fish in the boiling butter and poach it for 4 minutes.
5. Meanwhile, pour orange juice into the skillet. Add honey and bring the liquid to a boil.
6. Add cornstarch and whisk until the liquid will start to be thick.
7. Then remove it from the heat.
8. Transfer the poached halibut to the plate and cut it on 4.
9. Place every fish serving on the plate and top with orange sauce.

NUTRIENTS PER SERVING

- Calories: 349
- Protein: 17.8 g.
- Fat: 29.3 g.
- Carb: 3.2 g.
- Sodium: 167 mg.
- Potassium: 256 mg.
- Phosphorus: 236 mg.

44. Crazy Saganaki Shrimp

PREPARATION TIME
10’

COOK TIME
10’

SERVING
3

INGREDIENTS

- 12 jumbo shrimps, peeled and deveined with tails left on
- 1/2 cup Greek feta cheese, crumbled
- 1/2 cup Chardonnay
- 1 medium bulb fennel, cored and finely chopped
- 1 small chili pepper, seeded and minced
- 1 tbsp. extra virgin olive oil
- 2 tbsp. lemon juice, divided
- 5 scallions sliced thinly
- Pepper to taste
- 1/4 tsp. salt

DIRECTIONS

1. In a medium bowl, mix salt, lemon juice, and shrimp.
2. On medium fire, place a saganaki pan (or large nonstick saucepan) and heat oil.
3. Sauté chili pepper, scallions, and fennel for 4 minutes or until starting to brown and is already soft.
4. Add wine and sauté for another minute.
5. Place shrimps on top of the fennel, cover, and cook for 4 minutes or until shrimps are pink.
6. Remove just the shrimp and transfer to a plate.
7. Add pepper, feta, and 1 tbsp. lemon juice to pan and cook for a minute or until cheese begins to melt.
8. To serve, place cheese and fennel mixture on a serving plate and top with shrimps.

NUTRIENTS PER SERVING

- Calories: 310
- Protein: 49.7 g.
- Fat: 6.8 g.
- Carb: 8.4 g.
- Sodium: 121 mg.
- Potassium: 227 mg.
- Phosphorus: 316 mg.

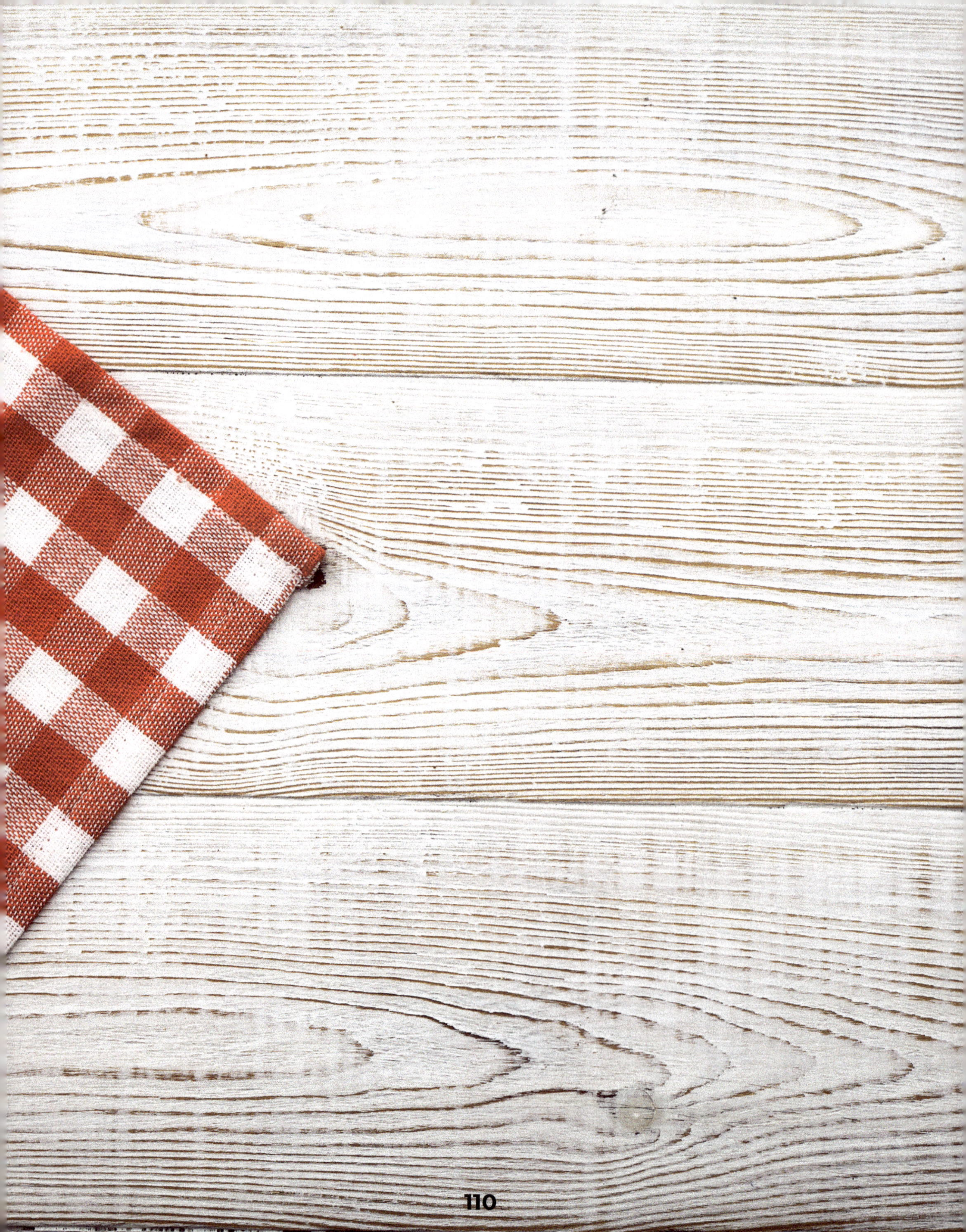

CHAPTER 14

Meat

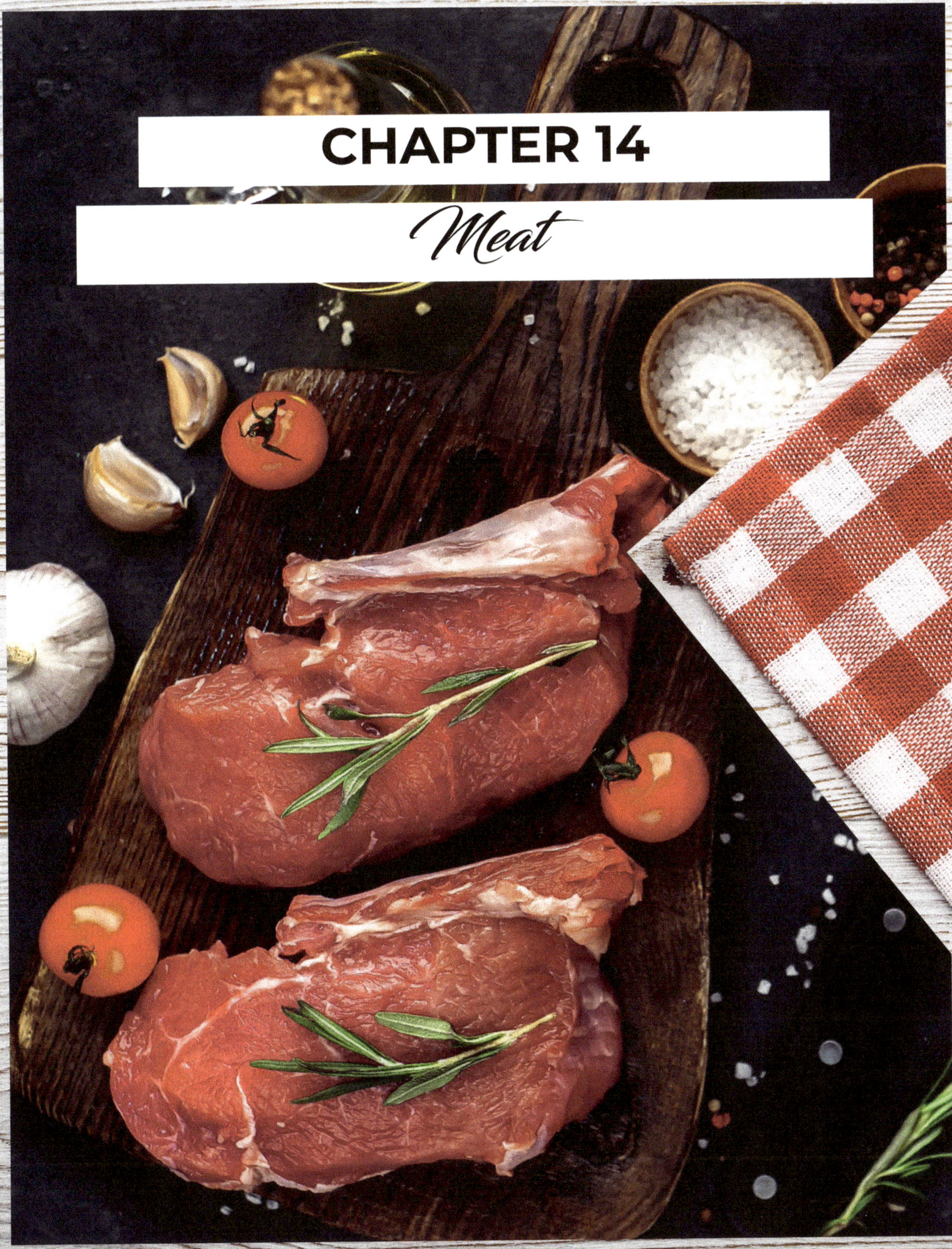

45. Peppercorn Pork Chops

PREPARATION TIME
20'

COOK TIME
25'

SERVING
4

INGREDIENTS

- 4 pork loin chops
- 1 tbsp. crushed black peppercorns
- 2 tbsp. olive oil
- 1/4 cup butter
- 5 garlic cloves
- 1 cup green and red bell peppers
- 1/2 cup pineapple juice

DIRECTIONS

1. Sprinkle and press peppercorns into both sides of pork chops.
2. Heat oil, butter, and garlic cloves in a large skillet over medium heat, stirring frequently.
3. Add pork chops and cook uncovered for 5–6 minutes.
4. Dice the bell peppers. Add the bell peppers and pineapple juice to the pork chops.
5. Cover and simmer for another 5–6 minutes or until pork is thoroughly cooked.

NUTRIENTS PER SERVING

- Calories: 317
- Protein: 13.2 g.
- Sodium: 126 mg.
- Potassium: 20 mg.
- Phosphorus: 115 mg.

46. Pork Chops With Apples

PREPARATION TIME
25'

COOK TIME
55'

SERVING
4

INGREDIENTS

- 4 pork chops
- Salt and pepper to taste
- 2 onions, sliced into rings
- 2 apples, peeled, cored, and sliced into rings
- 3 tbsp. honey
- 2 tsp. freshly ground black pepper

DIRECTIONS

1. Preheat oven to 375°F.
2. Spice pork chops with salt and pepper to taste, and arrange in a medium oven-safe skillet. Top pork chops with onions and apples. Sprinkle with honey. Season with 2 tsp. pepper.
3. Cover, and bake 1 hour in the preheated oven, pork chops have reached an internal temperature of 145°F.

NUTRIENTS PER SERVING

- Calories: 307
- Protein: 15 g.
- Sodium: 48 mg.
- Potassium: 387 mg.
- Phosphorus: 315 mg.

47. Beef Patties

PREPARATION TIME
10'

COOK TIME
8'

SERVING
4

INGREDIENTS

- 1 lb. ground beef
- 1 egg, lightly beaten
- 3 tbsp. almond flour
- 1 small onion, grated
- 2 tbsp. fresh parsley, chopped
- 1 tsp. dry oregano
- 1 tsp. dry mint
- Pepper
- Salt

DIRECTIONS

1. Mix all ingredients in a container till combined.
2. Make small patties from the meat mixture.
3. Heat grill pan over medium-high heat.
4. Place patties in a hot pan and cook for 4–5 minutes on each side.
5. Serve and enjoy.

NUTRIENTS PER SERVING

- Calories: 188
- Protein: 29 g.
- Fat: 6.6 g.
- Carb: 1.7 g.
- Sodium: 120 mg.
- Potassium: 227 mg.
- Phosphorus: 316 mg.

48. Roasted Sirloin Steak

PREPARATION TIME
10'

COOK TIME
30'

SERVING
6

INGREDIENTS

- 2 lb. sirloin steak, cut into 1" cubes
- 2 garlic cloves, minced
- 3 tbsp. fresh lemon juice
- 1 tsp. dried oregano
- 1/4 cup water
- 1/4 cup olive oil
- 2 cups fresh parsley, chopped
- 1/2 tsp. pepper
- 1 tsp. salt

DIRECTIONS

1. Add all ingredients except beef into the large bowl and mix well.
2. Pour bowl mixture into the large zip-lock bag.
3. Add beef to the bag and jiggle well and refrigerate for 1 hour.
4. Preheat the oven to 400°F.
5. Place marinated beef on a baking tray and bake in a preheated oven for 30 minutes.
6. Serve and enjoy.

NUTRIENTS PER SERVING

- Calories 365
- Protein: 46.6 g.
- Fat: 18.1 g.
- Carb: 2 g.
- Sodium: 178 g.
- Potassium: 204 mg.
- Phosphorus: 266 mg.

49. Classic Meatballs

PREPARATION TIME
10'

COOK TIME
4 HOURS

SERVING
6

INGREDIENTS

- 1/2 lb. ground beef
- 1/2 lb. ground pork
- 1 egg
- 2 tbsp. fresh parsley, chopped
- 1 garlic clove, minced
- 14 oz. can tomatoes, crushed
- 2 tbsp. fresh basil, chopped
- 1/4 tsp. pepper
- 1/2 tsp. salt

DIRECTIONS

1. In a mixing bowl, mix together beef, pork, egg, parsley, garlic, pepper, and salt until well combined.
2. Make small balls from the meat mixture.
3. Arrange meatballs into the slow cooker.
4. Pour crushed tomatoes, basil, pepper, and salt over meatballs.
5. Cover and cook on low for 4 hours.
6. Serve and enjoy.

NUTRIENTS PER SERVING

- Calories 150
- Protein: 24 g.
- Fat: 4 g.
- Carb: 4 g.
- Sodium: 134 mg.
- Potassium: 88 mg.
- Phosphorus: 76 mg.

50. Shredded Beef

PREPARATION TIME
10'

COOK TIME
5 H 10'

SERVING
4

INGREDIENTS

- 2 lb. beef rump roast
- 1/2 cup onion
- 2 garlic cloves
- 2 tbsp. fresh parsley
- 1 tbsp. Italian herb seasoning
- 1 tsp. dried parsley
- 1 bay leaf
- 1/2 tsp. pepper
- 1/4 tsp. salt
- 2 tbsp. olive oil
- 1/3 cup vinegar
- 2–3 cups of water
- 8 hard rolls, 3–1/2-inch diameter, 2 oz. each

DIRECTIONS

1. Chop onion, garlic, and fresh parsley. Place beef roast in a Crock-Pot. Add chopped onion, garlic, and remaining ingredients, except fresh parsley and rolls, to Crock-Pot; stir to combine.
2. Over low-heat setting, cover and cook for 8–10 hours, or on high setting for 4–5 hours, until fork-tender.
3. Remove roast from Crock-Pot.
4. Shred with two forks then return meat to cooking broth to keep warm until ready to serve.
5. Slice rolls in half and top with shredded beef, fresh parsley, and 1–2 spoons of the broth.
6. Serve open-face or as a sandwich.

NUTRIENTS PER SERVING

- Calories: 218
- Protein: 26 g.
- Sodium: 184 mg.
- Potassium: 28 mg.
- Phosphorus: 30 mg.

51. Lamb Stew With Green Beans

PREPARATION TIME
30'

COOK TIME
1 H 10'

SERVING
4

INGREDIENTS

- 1 lb. boneless lamb shoulder, cut into 2-inch pieces
- 1 tbsp. olive oil
- 1 large onion, chopped
- 1 stalk green onion, chopped
- 3 cups hot water
- 1/2 lb. fresh green beans, trimmed
- 1 tbsp. chopped fresh parsley
- 1/2 tsp. dried mint
- 1/2 tsp. dried dill weed
- 1 pinch ground nutmeg
- 1/4 tsp. honey
- Salt and pepper to taste

DIRECTIONS

1. In a large pot over moderate temperature, heat oil. Sauté onion and green onion until golden.
2. Stir in lamb, and cook until evenly brown.
3. Stir in water. Reduce heat and simmer for about 1 hour.
4. Stir in green beans. Season with parsley, mint, dill, nutmeg, honey, salt, and pepper.
5. Continue cooking until beans are tender.

NUTRIENTS PER SERVING

- Calories: 81
- Protein: 6.5 g.
- Sodium: 20 mg.
- Potassium: 136 mg.
- Phosphorus: 120 mg.

52. Laurel Lamb

PREPARATION TIME
5'

COOK TIME
30'

SERVING
4

INGREDIENTS

- 1.5 lb. lamb chops
- 3 cloves garlic
- 3 leaves laurel
- A sprig of oregano
- 2 tbsp. chopped parsley
- 1 tbsp. fresh or dried rosemary
- c/n virgin olive oil
- 1/3 cup vinegar
- 2–3 cups of water
- 8 hard rolls, 3–1/2-inch diameter, 2 oz. each

DIRECTIONS

1. Put the chops on a platter and sprinkle with herbs and garlic, peeled and chopped. Add salt and pepper and marinate overnight.
2. The next day put the meat in a bowl and sprinkle it with olive oil. Leave to marinate for at least 4 hours. Place all in a baking dish and close either with transparent foil.
3. Preheat the Airfryer to 282°F for 10 minutes.
4. Set the temperature to 338°F and leave about 15 minutes.
5. Now remove meat from the Airfryer and raise the temperature of the Airfryer to 428°F.
6. Remove the plastic wrap and return to the Airfryer for a few minutes until the meat has a golden color.
7. Serve with roasted or fried potatoes.

NUTRIENTS PER SERVING

- Calories: 206
- Protein: 13 g.
- Fat: 21.3 g.
- Carb: 15 g.
- Sodium: 129 mg.
- Potassium: 127 mg.
- Phosphorus: 216 mg.

53. Lamb Keema

PREPARATION TIME
10'

COOK TIME
15'

SERVING
4

INGREDIENTS

- 1 1/2 lb. ground lamb
- 1 onion, finely chopped
- 2 tsp. garlic powder
- 2 tbsp. garam masala
- 1/8 tsp. salt
- 3/4 cup chicken broth

DIRECTIONS

1. In a large, heavy skillet over average heat, cook ground lamb until evenly brown.
2. While cooking, break apart with a wooden spoon until crumbled.
3. Transfer cooked lamb to a bowl and drain off all but 1 tbsp. fat. Sauté onion until soft and translucent, about 5 minutes.
4. Stir in garlic powder, and sauté for 1 minute.
5. Stir in garam masala and cook for 1 minute.
6. Return the browned lamb to the pan, and stir in chicken beef broth.
7. Reduce heat, and simmer for 10–15 minutes or until meat is fully cooked through, and liquid has evaporated.

NUTRIENTS PER SERVING

- Calories: 194
- Protein: 28 g.
- Carb: 2.2 g.
- Sodium: 160 mg.
- Potassium: 379 mg.
- Phosphorus: 240 mg.

54. Beef With Red Kidney Beans

PREPARATION TIME
10'

COOK TIME
13'

SERVING
4

INGREDIENTS

- 12 oz. lean steak
- 1 onion, sliced
- 1 can chopped tomatoes
- 3/4 cup beef stock
- 4 tsp. fresh thyme, chopped
- 1 can red kidney beans
- Salt and pepper to taste
- Oven-safe bowl

DIRECTIONS

1. Preheat the air fryer oven to 390°F.
2. Set time to 13 minutes, cook for 3 minutes. Add the meat and continue cooking for 5 minutes.
3. Add the tomatoes and their juice, beef stock, thyme, and the beans and cook for an additional 5 minutes
4. Season with black pepper to taste.

NUTRIENTS PER SERVING

- Calories: 178
- Protein: 9 g.
- Fat: 14 g.
- Sodium: 131 mg.
- Potassium: 202 mg.
- Phosphorus: 116 mg.

55. Easy Pork Kabobs

PREPARATION TIME
10’

COOK TIME
4 H 20’

SERVING
6

INGREDIENTS

- 2 lb. pork tenderloin, cut into 1-inch cubes
- 1 onion, chopped
- 1/2 cup olive oil
- 1/2 cup red wine vinegar
- 2 tbsp. fresh parsley, chopped
- 2 garlic cloves, chopped
- Pepper
- Salt

DIRECTIONS

1. In a large zip-lock bag, mix red wine vinegar, parsley, garlic, onion, and oil.
2. Add meat to bag and marinate in the refrigerator overnight.
3. Remove marinated pork from the refrigerator and thread onto soaked wooden skewers. Season with pepper and salt.
4. Preheat the grill over high heat.
5. Grill pork for 3–4 minutes on both sides.
6. Serve and enjoy.

NUTRIENTS PER SERVING

- Calories: 375
- Protein: 40 g.
- Fat: 22 g.
- Carb: 2.5 g.
- Sodium: 129 mg.
- Potassium: 127 mg.
- Phosphorus: 136 mg.

56. Lamb Barley Soup

PREPARATION TIME
102

COOK TIME
60’

SERVING
4

INGREDIENTS

- 1 lb. ground lamb
- 1/2 large onion, chopped
- 2 cups of water
- 4 medium carrots, chopped
- 3 stalks celery, chopped
- 1/2 cup barley
- 1/2 tsp. chili powder
- 1/2 tsp. ground black pepper

DIRECTIONS

1. Heat a big skillet over medium-high warmth and stir in the ground lamb and onion.
2. Cook and stir until the lamb is evenly browned and onions are translucent.
3. Drain and discard any excess grease.
4. Add water, carrots, celery, and barley, and season with chili powder and pepper.
5. Simmer over medium heat for 45 minutes.

NUTRIENTS PER SERVING

- Calories: 79
- Protein: 4.8 g.
- Carb: 12.7 g.
- Sodium: 39 mg.
- Potassium: 221 mg.
- Phosphorus: 170 mg.

57. Feta Lamb Patties

PREPARATION TIME
10'

COOK TIME
12'

SERVING
4

INGREDIENTS

- 1 lb. ground lamb
- 1/2 tsp. garlic powder
- 1/2 cup feta cheese, crumbled
- 1/4 cup mint leaves, chopped
- 1/4 cup roasted red pepper, chopped
- 1/4 cup onion, chopped
- Pepper
- Salt

DIRECTIONS

1. Add all ingredients into the container and mix until well combined.
2. Spray pan with cooking spray and heat over medium-high heat.
3. Make small patties from meat mixture and place on a hot pan and cook for 6–7 minutes on each side.
4. Serve and enjoy.

NUTRIENTS PER SERVING

- Calories: 270
- Protein: 34.9 g.
- Fat: 12 g.
- Carb: 2.9 g.
- Sodium: 129 mg.
- Potassium: 137 mg.
- Phosphorus: 116 mg.

58. Simple Steak

PREPARATION TIME
6'

COOK TIME
14'

SERVING
2

INGREDIENTS

- 1/2 lb. quality cuts steak
- Salt and freshly ground black pepper, to taste

DIRECTIONS

1. Preheat the air fryer to 390°F.
2. Rub the steak with salt and pepper evenly.
3. Place the steak in the air fryer basket and cook for about 14 minutes until crispy.

NUTRIENTS PER SERVING

- Calories: 198
- Protein: 43 g.
- Fat: 7 g.
- Sodium: 131 mg.
- Potassium: 107 mg.
- Phosphorus: 126 mg.

CHAPTER 15

Poultry

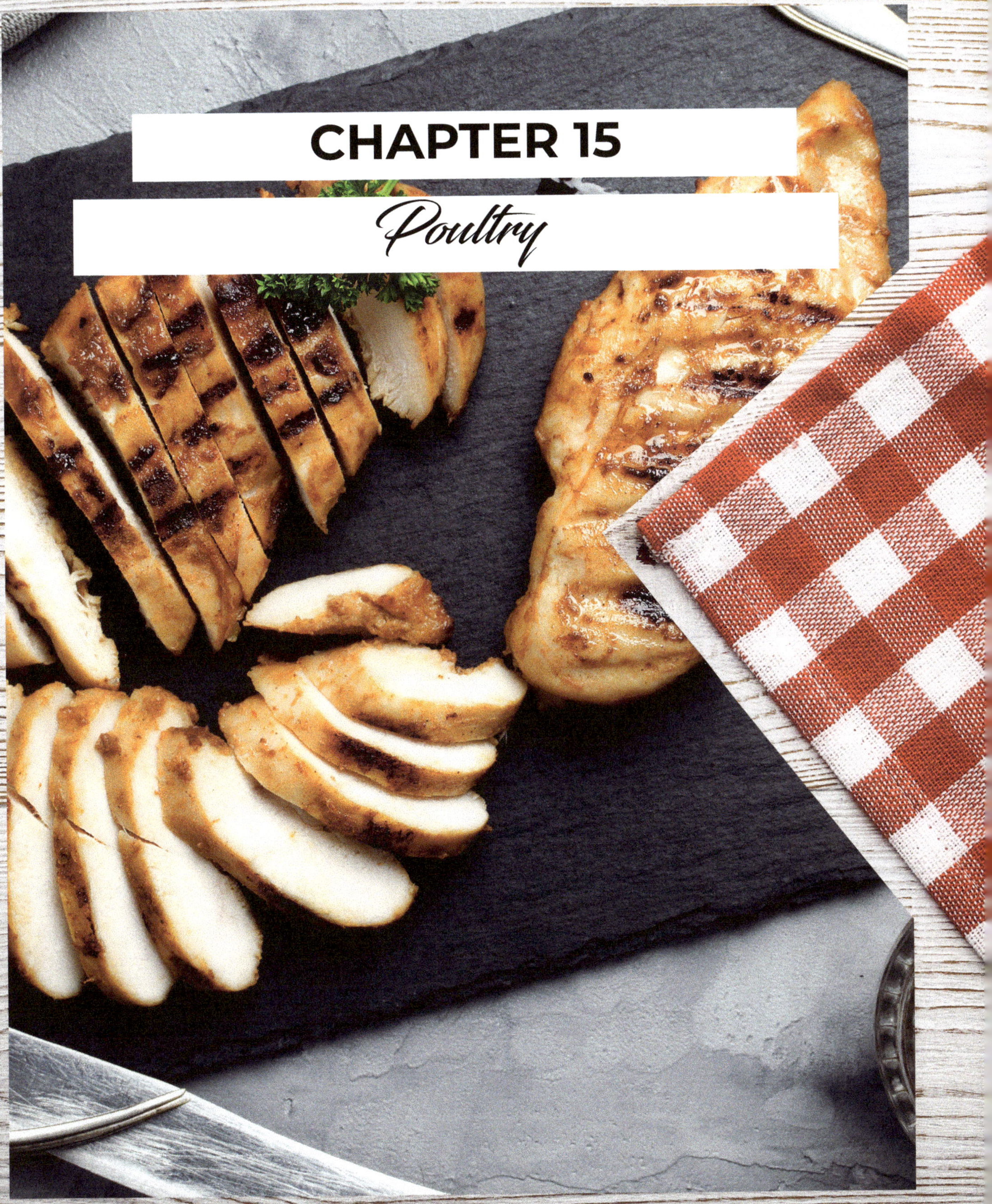

59. Creamy Turkey

PREPARATION TIME
12'

COOK TIME
10'

SERVING
4

INGREDIENTS

- 4 turkey breast halves, skinless, boneless
- 1/2 tsp. ground black pepper
- 1/2 tsp. garlic powder
- 1 (10.75 oz.) can chicken soup
- Salt and pepper to taste

DIRECTIONS

1. Preheat oven to 375°F.
2. Clean turkey breasts and season with salt, pepper, and garlic powder (or whichever seasonings you prefer) on both sides of turkey pieces.
3. Bake for 25 minutes, then add chicken soup and bake for 10 more minutes (or until done). Serve over rice or egg noodles.

NUTRIENTS PER SERVING

- Calories: 160
- Protein: 25.6 g.
- Sodium: 159 mg.
- Potassium: 152 mg.
- Phosphorus: 85 mg.

60. Lemon Pepper Chicken Legs

PREPARATION TIME
5’

COOK TIME
25’

SERVING
4

INGREDIENTS

- 8 chicken legs
- 1/2 tsp. garlic powder
- 2 tbsp. baking powder
- 4 tbsp. salted butter, melted
- 1 tbsp. lemon-pepper seasoning

DIRECTIONS

1. In a small container add the garlic powder and baking powder, then use this mixture to coat the chicken legs. Lay the chicken in the basket of your fryer.
2. Cook the chicken legs at 375°F for 25 minutes. Halfway through, turn them over and allow them to cook on the other side.
3. When the chicken has turned golden brown, test with a thermometer to ensure it has reached an ideal temperature of 165°F. Remove from the fryer.
4. Mix the melted butter and lemon pepper seasoning and toss with the chicken legs until the chicken is coated all over. Serve hot.

NUTRIENTS PER SERVING

- Calories: 132
- Protein: 48 g.
- Fat: 16 g.
- Carb: 20 g.
- Sodium: 125 mg.
- Potassium: 127 mg.
- Phosphorus: 132 mg.

61. Turkey Broccoli Salad

PREPARATION TIME
10'

COOK TIME
0'

SERVING
4

INGREDIENTS

- 3 turkey breast halves, cooked skinless, boneless cubed
- 8 cups broccoli florets
- 6 green onions, chopped
- 1 cup mayonnaise
- 1/4 cup apple cider vinegar
- 1/4 cup honey

DIRECTIONS

1. Combine broccoli, turkey, and green onions in a large bowl.
2. Whisk mayonnaise, vinegar, and honey together in a bowl until well blended.
3. Pour mayonnaise dressing over broccoli mixture; toss to coat.
4. Cover and refrigerate until chilled, if desired. Serve!

NUTRIENTS PER SERVING

- Calories 133
- Protein 6.2 g
- Sodium: 23 mg.
- Potassium: 150 mg.
- Phosphorus: 148 mg.

62. Fruity Chicken Salad

PREPARATION TIME
10'

COOK TIME
5'

SERVING
3

INGREDIENTS

- 4 chicken breast halves, skinless, boneless, cooked, and diced
- 1 stalk celery, diced
- 4 green onions, chopped
- 1 Golden Delicious apple, peeled, cored, and diced
- 1/3 cup green grapes, halved, seedless
- 1/8 tsp. ground black pepper
- 3/4 cup light mayonnaise

DIRECTIONS

1. In a large container, add the celery, chicken, onion, apple, grapes, pepper, and mayonnaise.
2. Mix all together. Serve!

NUTRIENTS PER SERVING

- Calories: 196
- Protein: 13.2 g.
- Carb: 15.6 g.
- Sodium: 180 mg.
- Potassium: 115 mg.
- Phosphorus: 88 mg.

63. Buckwheat Chicken Salad

PREPARATION TIME

12'

COOK TIME

20'

SERVING

3

INGREDIENTS

- 1 cup buckwheat, uncooked
- 2 large chicken breasts, cooked, cut into bite-size pieces
- 2 cups of water
- 1 clove garlic, smashed
- 1 large red onion, diced
- 1 large green bell pepper, diced
- 1/4 cup fresh parsley, chopped
- 1/4 cup fresh chives, chopped
- 1/2 tsp. salt
- 2/3 cup fresh lemon juice
- 1 tbsp. balsamic vinegar
- 1/4 cup olive oil

DIRECTIONS

1. Bring the water, garlic to a boil in a saucepan. Stir in the buckwheat, reduce heat to medium-low, cover, and simmer until the buckwheat is tender and the water has been absorbed, 15–20 minutes.
2. Discard the garlic clove and scrape the buckwheat into a large bowl.
3. Gently stir the chicken, onion, bell pepper, parsley, chives, and salt into the buckwheat.
4. Sprinkle with olive oil, balsamic vinegar, and lemon juice. Stir until evenly mixed.

NUTRIENTS PER SERVING

- Calories: 199
- Protein: 13.6 g.
- Fat: 8.3 g.
- Sodium: 108 mg.
- Potassium: 262 mg.
- Phosphorus: 188 mg.

64. Parmesan and Basil Turkey Salad

PREPARATION TIME
15'

COOK TIME
35'

SERVING
4

INGREDIENTS

- 2 whole turkey breasts, skinless, boneless
- 2/3 cup grated parmesan cheese
- Salt and pepper to taste
- 1 cup mayonnaise
- 1 cup chopped fresh basil
- 2 cloves crushed garlic
- 3 stalks celery, chopped

DIRECTIONS

1. Season turkey with salt and pepper. Roast at 375°F for 35 minutes, or until juices run clear. Let cool, and chop into chunks.
2. In a food processor, puree the mayonnaise, basil, garlic, and celery.
3. Combine the chunked turkey, puréed mixture, and parmesan cheese; toss.
4. Refrigerate, and serve.

NUTRIENTS PER SERVING

- Calories: 303
- Protein: 8.5 g.
- Sodium: 190 mg.
- Potassium: 121 mg.
- Phosphorus: 100 mg.

65. Healthy Chicken Nuggets

PREPARATION TIME
30'

COOK TIME
5 HOUS

SERVING
2 (5 NUGGETS PER SERVING)

INGREDIENTS

- 1 lb. chicken breast, cut into 1.5 inch
- 12 oz. Greek yogurt, low-fat/low-sodium
- 2 cup white flour
- 2 eggs, whisked
- 1 cup lemon juice
- 1/2 tbsp. garlic, minced
- 1/2 tbsp. lemon peel
- 1/2 black pepper, freshly ground
- c/n olive oil

DIRECTIONS

1. In a bowl mix the chicken with yogurt and lemon. Cover and put the container in the fridge, to marinate, minimum of 4 hours (better overnight)
2. When you're ready, preheat the oven to 400°F.
3. Take the chicken out of the fridge and let it come to room temperature. In three separate bowls: bowl 1: flour; bowl 2: whisked egg; bowl 3: crushed cornflake breadcrumbs mixed with spices.
4. Start dipping each strip or nugget into the flour, then dredge it in the egg, and finally rolling it in the cornflake crumbs. Place the nugget on an oiled baking sheet and put into the oven until brown and crispy, 15–20 minutes. Serve warm.

NUTRIENTS PER SERVING

- Calories 145
- Protein: 13.6 g.
- Fat: 2.3 g.
- Carb: 17 g.
- Sodium: 62 mg.
- Potassium: 149 mg.
- Phosphorus: 120 mg.

66. Honey Chicken Salad

PREPARATION TIME
5'

COOK TIME
15'

SERVING
4

INGREDIENTS

- 1 lb. chicken breast halves, skinless
- 1/2 tsp. dry mustard
- 1 tbsp. honey
- 2 green onions, chopped
- 1/2 cup mayonnaise
- 1 tsp. apple cider vinegar

DIRECTIONS

1. Boil water in a large pot. Add the chicken and simmer until cooked thoroughly approximately 10 minutes. Drain, cool, and cut into cubes.
2. In a large bowl toss together mayonnaise, dry mustard, honey, onions, and vinegar.
3. Add chicken. Stir until evenly coated, adding more mayonnaise if necessary. Refrigerate until serving.

NUTRIENTS PER SERVING

- Calories 280
- Protein: 25 g.
- Fat: 19 g.
- Carb: 6 g.
- Sodium: 220 mg.
- Potassium: 240 mg.
- Phosphorus: 198 mg.

67. Oven-Baked Turkey Thighs

PREPARATION TIME
10'

COOK TIME
30'

SERVING
4

INGREDIENTS

- 10 oz. turkey thighs, skin on, bone-in
- 1/3 cup white wine
- 1 lemon
- 1 tbsp. fresh oregano
- 1/4 tsp. cracked black pepper
- 1 tbsp. olive oil

DIRECTIONS

1. Heat the oven to 350°F.
2. Add turkey thighs and white wine to an oven-proof pan. Squeeze half the lemon over the turkey. Slice remaining lemon and top turkey with lemon slices.
3. Season turkey with fresh oregano, cracked pepper, and olive oil.
4. Bake turkey for 25–30 minutes or until internal temperature reaches 165–175°F.

NUTRIENTS PER SERVING

- Calories: 189
- Protein: 20.8 g.
- Sodium: 62 mg.
- Potassium: 232 mg.
- Phosphorus: 180 mg.

68. Southern Fried Chicken

PREPARATION TIME

5'

COOK TIME

26'

SERVING

2

INGREDIENTS

- 2–6 oz. chicken breasts, boneless, skinless.
- 2 tbsp. hot sauce
- 1/2 tsp. onion powder
- 1 tbsp. chili powder
- 2 oz. pork rinds, finely ground

DIRECTIONS

1. Chop the chicken breasts in half lengthways and rub in the hot sauce. Combine the onion powder with the chili powder, then rub it into the chicken. Leave to marinate for at least a 1/2 hour.
2. Use the ground pork rinds to coat the chicken breasts in the ground pork rinds, covering them thoroughly. Place the chicken in your fryer.
3. Set the fryer at 350°F and cook the chicken for 13 minutes. Turn over the chicken and cook the other side for another 13 minutes or until golden.
4. Test the chicken with a meat thermometer. When fully cooked, it should reach 165°F. Serve hot, with the sides of your choice.

NUTRIENTS PER SERVING

- Calories: 408
- Protein: 35 g.
- Fat: 19 g.
- Carb: 10 g.
- Phosphorus: 216 mg.
- Potassium: 137 mg.
- Sodium: 153 mg.

69. Cilantro Drumsticks

PREPARATION TIME
12'

COOK TIME
18'

SERVING
4

INGREDIENTS

- 8 chicken drumsticks
- 1/2 cup chimichurri sauce
- 1/4 cup lemon juice

DIRECTIONS

1. Coat the chicken drumsticks with chimichurri sauce and refrigerate in an airtight container for no less than 1 hour, ideally overnight.
2. When it's time to cook, pre-heat your fryer to 400°F.
3. Remove the chicken from the refrigerator and allow return to room temperature for roughly 20 minutes.
4. Cook for 18 minutes in the fryer. Drizzle with lemon juice to taste and enjoy.

NUTRIENTS PER SERVING

- Calories: 470
- Protein: 36 g.
- Fat: 29 g.
- Carb: 16 g.
- Sodium: 123 mg.
- Potassium: 227 mg.
- Phosphorus 146 mg.

70. Basil Chicken Over Macaroni

PREPARATION TIME
10'

COOK TIME
30'

SERVING
4

INGREDIENTS

- 1 (8 oz.) package macaroni
- 2 tsp. olive oil
- 1/2 cup finely chopped onion
- 1 clove garlic, chopped
- 2 cups chicken breast halves, boneless, cooked, and cubed
- 1/4 cup fresh basil, chopped
- 1/4 cup parmesan cheese
- 1/2 tsp. black pepper

DIRECTIONS

1. In a large pot of boiling water, cook macaroni until it is al dente, about 8–10 minutes. Drain, and set aside.
2. In a large skillet, heat oil over medium-high heat. Sauté the onions and garlic. Stir in the chicken, basil, and pepper.
3. Reduce heat to medium, and cover skillet. Simmer for about 5 minutes, stirring frequently,
4. Toss sauce with hot cooked macaroni to coat. Serve with parmesan cheese.

NUTRIENTS PER SERVING

- Calories: 349
- Protein: 28.5 g.
- Sodium: 65 mg.
- Potassium: 286 mg.
- Phosphorus: 280 mg.

71. Chicken Sauté

PREPARATION TIME

10'

COOK TIME

25'

SERVING

2

INGREDIENTS

- 4 oz. chicken fillet
- 4 tomatoes, peeled
- 1 bell pepper, chopped
- 1 tsp. olive oil
- 1 cup of water
- 1 tsp. salt
- 1 chili pepper, chopped
- 1/2 tsp. saffron

DIRECTIONS

1. Pour water into the pan and bring it to a boil.
2. Meanwhile, chop the chicken fillet.
3. Add the chicken fillet to the boiling water and cook it for 10 minutes or until the chicken is tender.
4. After this, put the chopped bell pepper and chili pepper in the skillet.
5. Add olive oil and roast the vegetables for 3 minutes.
6. Add chopped tomatoes and mix up well.
7. Cook the vegetables for 2 minutes more.
8. Then add salt and a 3/4 cup of water from the chicken.
9. Add chopped chicken fillet and mix up.
10. Cook the sauté for 10 minutes over medium heat.

NUTRIENTS PER SERVING

- Calories 192
- Protein: 19.3 g.
- Fat: 7.2 g.
- Carb: 14.4 g.
- Sodium: 101 mg.
- Potassium: 227 mg.
- Phosphorus: 216 mg.

72. Grilled Marinated Chicken

PREPARATION TIME
35'

COOK TIME
20'

SERVING
6

INGREDIENTS

- 2 lb. chicken breast, skinless, boneless
- 2 tbsp. lemon juice
- 1 tsp. sage
- 1/2 tsp. ground nutmeg
- 1/2 tsp. dried oregano
- 1 tsp. paprika
- 1 tsp. onion powder
- 2 tbsp. olive oil
- 1 tsp. chili flakes
- 1 tsp. salt
- 1 tsp. apple cider vinegar

DIRECTIONS

1. Make the marinade: whisk together apple cider vinegar, salt, chili flakes, olive oil, onion powder, paprika, dried oregano, ground nutmeg, sage, and lemon juice.
2. Then rub the chicken with marinade carefully and leave for 25 minutes to marinate.
3. Meanwhile, preheat the grill to 385°F.
4. Place the marinated chicken breast in the grill and cook it for 10 minutes from each side.
5. Cut the cooked chicken on the servings.

NUTRIENTS PER SERVING

- Calories: 218
- Protein: 32.3 g.
- Fat 8.2 g.
- Carb: 0.4 g.
- Sodium: 123 mg.
- Potassium: 207 mg.
- Phosphorus: 116 mg.

73. Tasty Turkey Patties

PREPARATION TIME
10'

COOK TIME
12'

SERVING
4

INGREDIENTS

- 14.5 oz. turkey
- 1 oz. cream cheese
- 1 large egg
- 1/8 tsp. ground sage
- 1/2 tsp. garlic powder
- 1/2 tsp. black pepper
- 1 tsp. onion powder
- 1 tsp. Italian seasoning
- 3/4 cup graham crackers crumbs
- 3 tbsp. olive oil

DIRECTIONS

1. Set cream cheese out to soften.
2. Using a fork, mash turkey with juices in a medium bowl.
3. Add the cream cheese, egg, sage, garlic powder, black pepper, onion powder, Italian seasoning, and graham crackers crumbs; mix well.
4. Form 4 patties.
5. Heat olive oil on low hotness, in a small skillet.
6. Fry patties for 5–6 minutes on each side or until crispy on the outside and heated thoroughly.

NUTRIENTS PER SERVING

- Calories: 270
- Protein: 13.5 g.
- Sodium: 204 mg.
- Potassium: 143 mg.
- Phosphorus: 100 mg.

CHAPTER 16

Vegetables

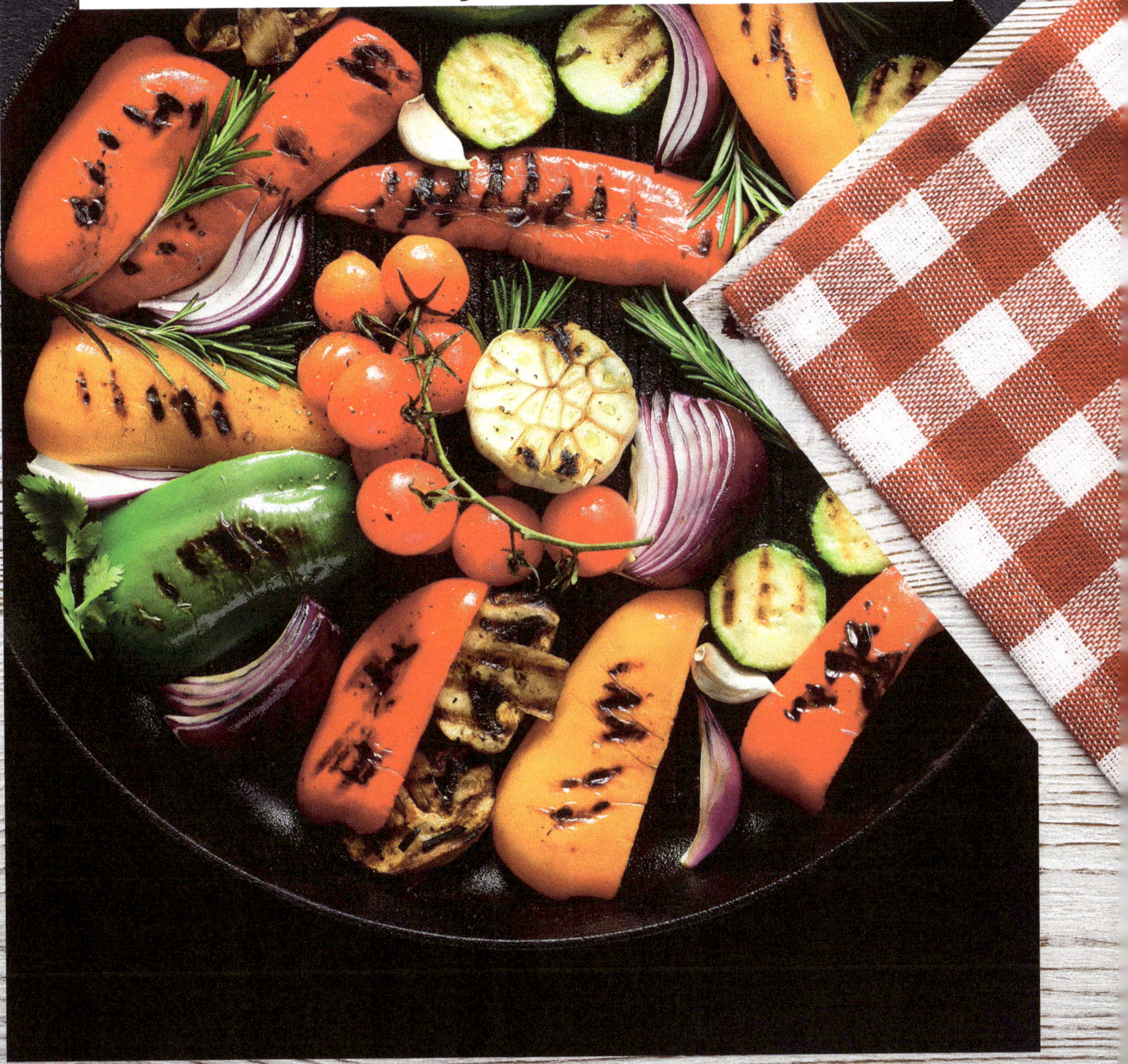

74. Thai Tofu Broth

PREPARATION TIME
5'

COOK TIME
15'

SERVING
4

INGREDIENTS

- 1 cup of rice noodles
- 1/2 onion, sliced
- 6 oz. tofu, pressed and cubed, drained
- 1/4 cup scallions, sliced
- 1/2 cup water
- 1/2 cup canned water chestnuts
- 1/2 cup rice milk
- 1 tbsp. lime juice
- 1 tbsp. coconut oil
- 1/2 chili, finely sliced
- 1 cup snow peas

DIRECTIONS

1. Warm the oil in a wok at a high temperature and then sauté the tofu until brown on each side.
2. Add the onion and sauté for 2–3 minutes.
3. Add the rice milk and water to the wok until bubbling.
4. Lower to medium heat and add the noodles, chili, and water chestnuts.
5. Allow to simmer for 10–15 minutes and then add the sugar snap peas for 5 minutes.
6. Serve with a sprinkle of scallions.

NUTRIENTS PER SERVING

- Calories: 304
- Protein: 9 g.
- Fat: 13 g.
- Sodium: 36 mg.
- Potassium: 114 mg.
- Phosphorus: 101 mg.

75. Delicious Vegetarian Lasagna

PREPARATION TIME
10'

COOK TIME
1 HOUR

SERVING
2

INGREDIENTS

- 3 lasagna sheets
- 1 tsp. basil
- 1 tbsp. olive oil
- 1/2 red pepper, sliced
- 1/2 red onion, diced
- 1/4 tsp. black pepper
- 1 cup of rice milk
- 1 garlic clove, minced
- 1 cup eggplant, sliced
- 1/2 zucchini, sliced
- 1/2 pack soft tofu
- 1 tsp. oregano

DIRECTIONS

1. Turn on the oven to 325°F.
2. Slice zucchini, eggplant, and pepper into vertical strips.
3. Add the rice milk and tofu to a food processor and blitz until smooth. Set aside.
4. Heat the oil in a skillet over average heat, add the onions, and garlic for 3–4 minutes or until soft.
5. Sprinkle in the herbs and pepper and allow to stir through for 5–6 minutes until hot.
6. Into a lasagna or suitable oven dish, layer 1 lasagna sheet, then 1/3 the eggplant, followed by 1/3 zucchini, then 1/3 pepper before pouring over 1/3 of tofu white sauce.
7. Repeat for the next 2 layers, finishing with the white sauce.
8. Add to the oven for 40–50 minutes or until veg is soft and can easily be sliced into servings.

NUTRIENTS PER SERVING

- Calories: 470
- Protein: 10 g.
- Fat: 18 g.
- Sodium: 80 mg.
- Potassium: 260 mg.
- Phosphorus: 132 mg.

76. Chili Tofu Noodles

PREPARATION TIME
5'

COOK TIME
15'

SERVING
4

INGREDIENTS

- 2 cups of rice noodles
- 1/2 red chili, diced
- 1/2 juiced lime
- 6 oz. tofu, pressed and cubed silken firm
- 1 tsp. fresh ginger, grated
- 1 tbsp. coconut oil
- 1 cup green beans
- 1 garlic clove, minced

DIRECTIONS

1. Steam the green beans for 10–12 minutes or according to package directions and drain.
2. Cook the noodles in a pot of boiling water for 10–15 minutes, or according to package directions.
3. Meanwhile, heat a wok or skillet on high heat and add coconut oil.
4. Now add the tofu, chili flakes, garlic, and ginger. Sauté for 5–10 minutes.
5. Strain noodles and add to the wok along with the green beans and lime juice.
6. Toss to coat.
7. Serve hot!

NUTRIENTS PER SERVING

- Calories: 246
- Protein: 10 g.
- Fat: 12 g.
- Sodium: 25 mg.
- Potassium: 126 mg.
- Phosphorus: 79 mg.

77. Curried Cauliflower

PREPARATION TIME
5'

COOK TIME
20'

SERVING
4

INGREDIENTS

- 2 cups cauliflower florets
- 1 tsp. turmeric
- 1 onion, diced
- 1 tbsp. fresh cilantro, chopped
- 1 tsp. cumin
- 1/2 chili, diced
- 1/2 cup water
- 1 garlic clove, minced
- 1 tbsp. coconut oil
- 1 tsp. garam masala

DIRECTIONS

1. Add the oil to a skillet on average heat.
2. Sauté the onion and garlic for 5 minutes until soft.
3. Add the cumin, turmeric, and garam masala, stir to release the aromas.
4. Now add the chili to the pan along with the cauliflower.
5. Stir to coat.
6. Pour in the water and reduce the heat to a simmer for 15 minutes.
7. Garnish with cilantro to serve.

NUTRIENTS PER SERVING

- Calories: 108
- Protein: 2 g.
- Fat: 7 g.
- Sodium: 35 mg.
- Potassium: 328 mg.
- Phosphorus: 39 mg.

78. Chinese Tempeh Stir Fry

PREPARATION TIME
5'

COOK TIME
15'

SERVING
2

INGREDIENTS

- 2 oz. tempeh, sliced
- 1 cup brown rice, cooked
- 1 garlic clove, minced
- 1/2 cup green onions
- 1 tsp. fresh ginger, minced
- 1 tbsp. coconut oil
- 1/2 cup corn

DIRECTIONS

1. Heat the oil in a skillet or wok on high heat and add the garlic and ginger.
2. Sauté for 1 minute.
3. Now add the tempeh and cook for 5–6 minutes before adding the corn, cook further for 10 minutes.
4. Now add the green onions and serve over brown rice.

NUTRIENTS PER SERVING

- Calories: 304
- Protein: 10 g.
- Fat: 4 g.
- Sodium: 91 mg.
- Potassium: 121 mg.
- Phosphorus: 222 mg.

79. Parsley Root Veg Stew

PREPARATION TIME

5’

COOK TIME

35-40’

SERVING

4

INGREDIENTS

- 2 cups white rice
- 2 garlic cloves
- 1 tsp. ground cumin
- 1 onion, diced
- 2 cups of water
- 4 turnips, peeled and diced
- 1 tsp. cayenne pepper
- 1/4 cup fresh parsley, chopped
- 1/2 tsp. ground cinnamon
- 2 tbsp. olive oil
- 1 tsp. ground ginger
- 2 carrots, peeled and diced

DIRECTIONS

1. In a large pot, heat oil above medium-high heat before sautéing the onion for 4–5 minutes until soft.
2. Add the turnips and cook for 10 minutes or until golden brown.
3. Add the garlic, cumin, ginger, cinnamon, and cayenne pepper, cooking for a further 3 minutes.
4. Add the carrots and stock to the pot and then bring to the boil.
5. Turn the heat down to medium heat, cover, and simmer for 20 minutes.
6. Meanwhile, add the rice to a pot of water and bring to boil.
7. Turn down to simmer for 15 minutes.
8. Drain and place the lid on for 5 minutes to steam.
9. Garnish the root vegetable stew with parsley to serve alongside the rice.

NUTRIENTS PER SERVING

- Calories: 210
- Protein: 4 g.
- Fat: 7 g.
- Sodium: 67 mg.
- Potassium: 181 mg.
- Phosphorus: 105 mg.

80. Mixed Pepper Paella

PREPARATION TIME

10’

COOK TIME

35-40’

SERVING

2

INGREDIENTS

- 1 cup of brown rice
- 1 tbsp. extra-virgin olive oil
- 1/2 red onion, chopped
- 1 lemon
- 1/2 yellow bell pepper, chopped
- 1 cup homemade chicken broth
- 1/2 zucchini, chopped
- 1 tsp. dried oregano
- 1/2 red bell pepper, chopped
- 1 tsp. dried parsley
- 1 tsp. paprika

DIRECTIONS

1. In a pot of cold water, add rice, and cook for 15 minutes.
2. Drain the water, cover the pan, and leave to one side.
3. Heat the oil in a skillet over medium-high heat.
4. Add the bell peppers, onion, and zucchini, sautéing for 5 minutes.
5. To the pan, add the rice, herbs, spices, and juice of the lemon along with the chicken broth.
6. Shield and turn the heat right down and allow to simmer for 15–20 minutes.
7. Serve hot.

NUTRIENTS PER SERVING

- Calories: 210
- Protein: 4 g.
- Fat: 7 g.
- Sodium: 20 mg.
- Potassium: 33 mg.
- Phosphorus: 156 mg.

81. Minted Zucchini Noodles

PREPARATION TIME
5'

COOK TIME
10'

SERVING
2

INGREDIENTS

- 4 zucchinis, peeled and sliced
- 1/4 red chili, deseeded and chopped
- 2 tbsp. extra virgin olive oil
- 1/2 juiced lemon
- 1/2 cup fresh mint, chopped
- 1 tsp. black pepper
- 1/2 cup arugula

DIRECTIONS

1. Whisk the mint, pepper, chili, and olive oil to make a dressing.
2. Meanwhile, heat a pan of water on high heat and bring to a boil.
3. Add the zucchini noodles and turn the heat down to simmer for 3–4 minutes.
4. Remove from the heat and place in a bowl of cold water immediately.
5. Toss the noodles in the dressing.
6. Mix the arugula with the lemon juice to serve on the top. Enjoy!

NUTRIENTS PER SERVING

- Calories: 148
- Protein: 2 g.
- Fat: 13 g.
- Sodium: 7 mg.
- Potassium: 422 mg.
- Phosphorus: 256 mg.

82. Vegan Lasagna

PREPARATION TIME
10'

COOK TIME
1 HOUR

SERVING
3

INGREDIENTS

- 1/2 pack of soft tofu
- 1 garlic clove, crushed
- 4 tbsp. of rice milk (unenriched)
- 2 tbsp. of fresh basil, chopped
- 1 lemon, juiced
- A pinch of black pepper to taste
- 1/2 cup baby spinach
- 1 zucchini, sliced
- 1 red bell pepper, sliced
- 1 eggplant, sliced

DIRECTIONS

1. Preheat oven to 325°F (170°C) and soak vegetables in warm water before cooking.
2. In a blender, process the tofu, garlic, milk, basil, lemon juice, and pepper until smooth.
3. Toss in the spinach and zucchini for the last 30 seconds.
4. Layer the bottom of the dish with 1/3 the eggplant slices and 1/3 red pepper slices and then cover with 1/3 of the tofu sauce.
5. Repeat for a second layer.
6. Repeat for a third layer.
7. Bake in the oven for 1 hour or until the vegetables are soft through to the center (use your knife to test the middle).
8. Finish under the broiler until golden and bubbly.
9. Divide into portions and serve with a sprinkle of black pepper to taste.

NUTRIENTS PER SERVING

- Calories: 91
- Protein: 6 g.
- Fat: 3 g.
- Carb: 12 g.
- Sodium: 21 mg.
- Potassium: 368 mg.
- Phosphorus: 110 mg.

83. Zucchini Garlic Fries

PREPARATION TIME
10'

COOK TIME
20'

SERVING
6

INGREDIENTS

- 1/4 tsp. garlic powder
- 1/2 cup almond flour
- 2 large egg whites, beaten
- 3 medium zucchinis, sliced into fry sticks
- Salt and pepper to taste

DIRECTIONS

1. Preheat oven to 400°F.
2. Mix all ingredients in a bowl until the zucchini fries are well coated.
3. Place fries on a cookie sheet and spread evenly.
4. Put in oven and cook for 20 minutes.
5. Halfway through cooking time, stir-fries.

NUTRIENTS PER SERVING

- Calories: 110
- Protein: 1.5 g.
- Sodium: 19 mg.
- Potassium: 71 mg.
- Phosphorus: 116 mg.

84. Mashed Cauliflower

PREPARATION TIME
10'

COOK TIME
10'

SERVING
3

INGREDIENTS

- 1 cauliflower head
- 1 tbsp. olive oil
- 1/2 tsp. salt
- 1/4 tsp. dill
- Pepper to taste
- 2 tbsp. low-fat milk

DIRECTIONS

1. Boil water in a small pot.
2. Chop cauliflower in florets.
3. Add florets to boiling water and boil uncovered for 5 minutes. Turn off the fire and let it sit for 5 minutes more.
4. In a blender, add all ingredients except for cauliflower and blend to mix well.
5. Drain cauliflower well and add it into the blender. Puree until smooth and creamy.

NUTRIENTS PER SERVING

- Calories: 78
- Protein: 2 g.
- Sodium: 420 mg.
- Potassium: 327 mg.
- Phosphorus: 126 mg.

85. Brie, Chive and Scallion Tart

PREPARATION TIME
10'

COOK TIME
50'

SERVING
4

INGREDIENTS

For the pastry:

- 1 cup all-purpose white flour
- 1/2 cup unsalted butter, cubed
- 1/4 cup rice milk, unenriched

For the filling:

- 1 egg
- 1 egg yolk
- 1 cup rice milk, unenriched
- 1 tsp. black pepper
- 2 stems of scallion, chopped
- 1/2 cup brie cheese
- 1 tbsp. chives, finely chopped
- Approx. 10 cm. tart tin
- Baking beads
- Foil

DIRECTIONS

1. Sift the flour and add the butter by rubbing with fingers to create a breadcrumb texture.
2. Mix in the milk for the pastry slowly to bind and then knead on a work surface into a ball shape.
3. Wrap dough in plastic wrap and add to the fridge to cool.
4. Preheat the oven to 350°F (180°C).
5. Lightly flour the work surface and use a rolling pin to roll the pastry to approx. 1 cm. thick.
6. Gently use your fingers to lift the pastry over the base of the tart tin.
7. Line the pastry with the foil followed by the baking beads and add to the oven for 15 minutes.
8. Now trim the edges of the pastry from around the pastry tin.
9. Remove beads and foil and score the pastry with a fork before adding back into the oven for a further 15 minutes or until starting to turn golden.
10. While the pastry is cooking prepare the filling by beating the egg, egg yolk, and milk in a separate bowl and seasoning with pepper.
11. Add the chopped scallions, crumbled brie, and chopped chives to this mixture and gently pour into the pastry base.
12. Bake in the oven for 35 minutes or until cooked through and golden.
13. Serve warm.

NUTRIENTS PER SERVING

- Calories: 456
- Protein: 11 g.
- Fat: 33 g.
- Carb: 29 g.
- Sodium: 208 mg.
- Potassium: 198 mg.
- Phosphorus: 147 mg.

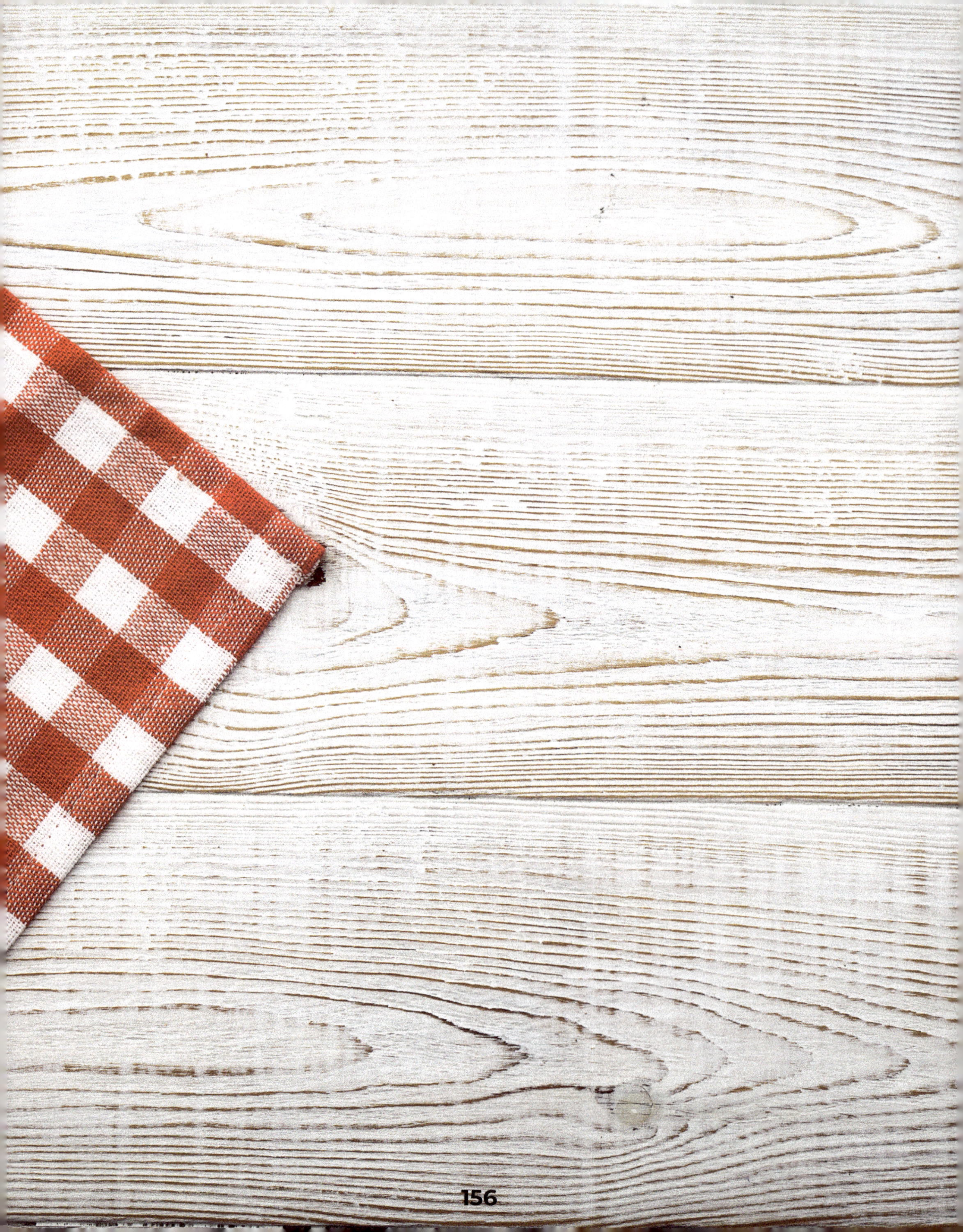

CHAPTER 17

Salads

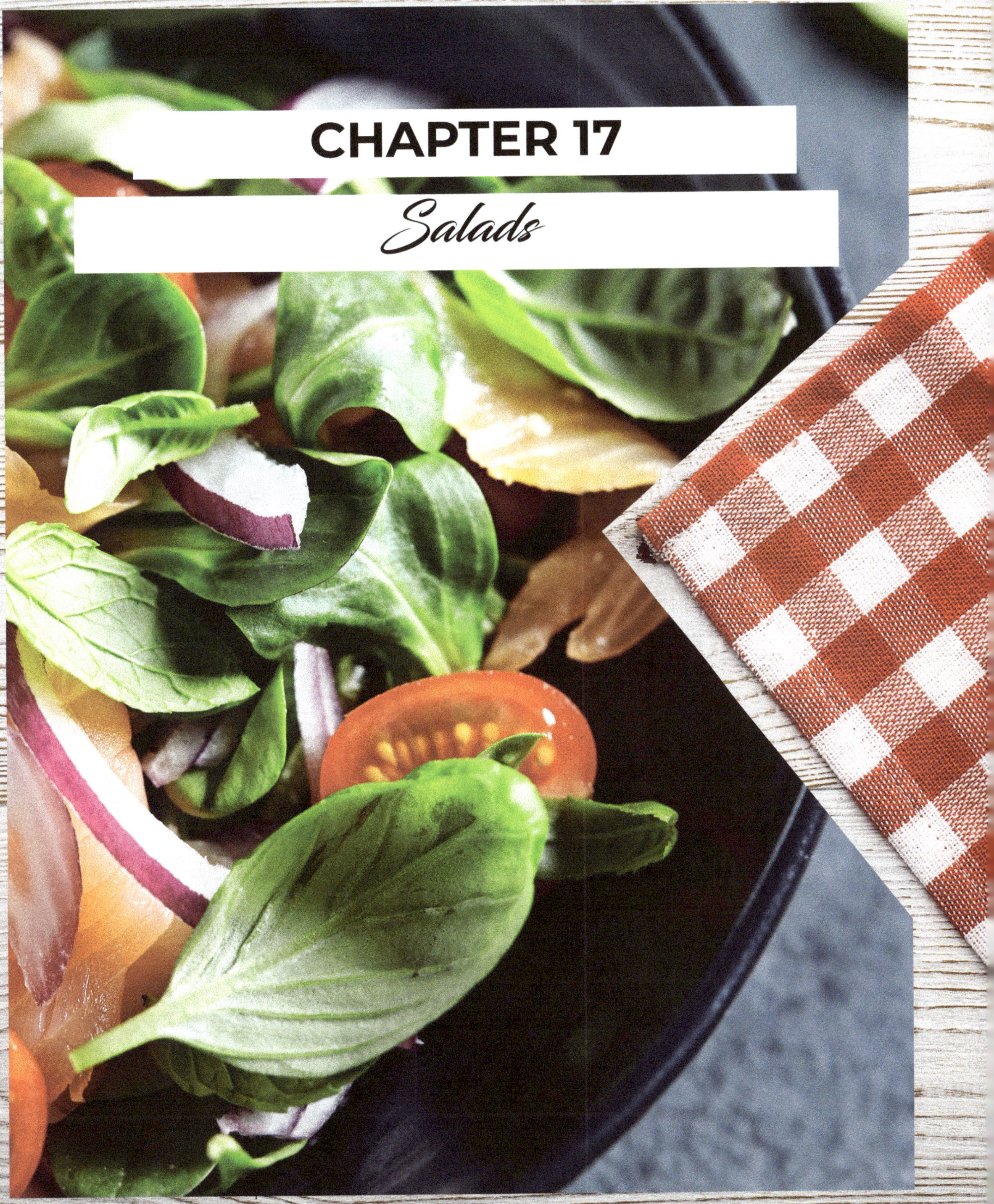

86. Pear & Brie Salad

PREPARATION TIME
5'

COOK TIME
0'

SERVING
4

INGREDIENTS

- 1 tbsp. olive oil
- 1 cup arugula
- 1/2 lemon
- 1/2 cup canned pears
- 1/4 cucumber
- 1/4 cup brie cheese, chopped

DIRECTIONS

1. Peel and dice the cucumber.
2. Dice the pear.
3. Wash the arugula.
4. Combine salad in a serving bowl and crumble the brie over the top.
5. Whisk the olive oil and lemon juice together.
6. Drizzle over the salad.
7. Season with a little black pepper to taste and serve immediately.

NUTRIENTS PER SERVING

- Calories: 54
- Protein: 1 g.
- Fat: 7 g.
- Carb: 12 g.
- Sodium: 57 mg.
- Potassium: 115 mg.
- Phosphorus: 67 mg.

87. Caesar Salad

PREPARATION TIME
5'

COOK TIME
5'

SERVING
4

INGREDIENTS

- 1 head romaine lettuce
- 1/4 cup mayonnaise
- 1 tbsp. lemon juice
- 4 anchovy fillets
- 1 tsp. Worcestershire sauce
- Black pepper
- 5 garlic cloves
- 4 tbsp. parmesan cheese
- 1 tsp. mustard

DIRECTIONS

1. In a bowl mix all ingredients and mix well
2. Serve with dressing

NUTRIENTS PER SERVING

- Calories: 44
- Protein: 3.2 g.
- Fat: 2.1 g.
- Carb: 4.3 g.
- Sodium: 83 mg.
- Potassium: 27 mg.
- Phosphorus: 45.6 mg.

88. Delicious Cucumber Salad

PREPARATION TIME
10'

COOK TIME
0'

SERVING
2

INGREDIENTS

- 2 cucumbers
- 1 tbsp. white sugar
- 1/2 cup cilantro
- 1 tbsp. white wine vinegar, or lemon juice
- 1/3 cup sour cream
- 1/8 cup black pepper

DIRECTIONS

1. Slice cucumbers and add all ingredients in a small basin and combine well.
2. Chill before serving.

NUTRIENTS PER SERVING

- Calories: 96
- Protein: 1 g.
- Fat: 6 g.
- Carb: 10 g.
- Sodium: 28 mg.
- Potassium: 125 mg.
- Phosphorus: 48 mg.

89. Barb's Asian Slaw

PREPARATION TIME
5'

COOK TIME
5'

SERVING
2

INGREDIENTS

- 1 cabbage head, shredded
- 4 chopped green onions
- 1/2 cup slivered or sliced almonds

Dressing:

- 1/2 cup olive oil
- 1/4 cup tamari or soy sauce
- 1 tbsp. honey or maple syrup
- 1 tbsp. baking stevia

DIRECTIONS

1. Heat up dressing ingredients in a saucepan on the stove until thoroughly mixed.
2. Mix all ingredients when you are ready to serve.

NUTRIENTS PER SERVING

- Calories: 205
- Protein: 27 g.
- Fat: 10 g.
- Carb: 12 g.
- Sodium: 110 mg.
- Potassium: 27 mg.
- Phosphorus: 76 mg.

90. Tarragon and Pepper Pasta

PREPARATION TIME
10'

COOK TIME
35'

SERVING
4

INGREDIENTS

- 2 cups white pasta
- 1 red bell pepper, finely diced
- 1/2 cucumber, finely diced
- 1/4 red onion, finely sliced
- 1 tsp. black pepper
- 2 tbsp. extra virgin olive oil
- 1 tbsp. dried tarragon

DIRECTIONS

1. Bring a pan of water to the boil before adding pasta for 15–20 minutes or according to package directions.
2. Drain and allow the pasta to cool before combining the rest of the raw ingredients and mixing well.
3. Serve right away or cover and refrigerate for 2–3 days.

NUTRIENTS PER SERVING

- Calories: 156
- Protein: 4 g.
- Fat: 7 g.
- Carb: 20 g.
- Sodium: 2 mg.
- Potassium: 147 mg.
- Phosphorus: 46 mg.

91. Italian Cucumber Salad

PREPARATION TIME
5'

COOK TIME
0'

SERVING
2

INGREDIENTS

- 2 cucumbers, sliced
- 1/4 cup rice vinegar
- 1/8 tsp. stevia
- 1 tsp. olive oil
- 1/8 tsp. black pepper
- 1 cup carrots, sliced
- 2 tbsp. green onion, sliced
- 2 tbsp. red bell pepper, sliced
- 1/2 tsp. Italian seasoning blend

DIRECTIONS

1. Put all the salad ingredients into a suitable salad bowl.
2. Toss them well and refrigerate for 1 hour.
3. Serve!

NUTRIENTS PER SERVING

- Calories: 112
- Fat: 1.6 g.
- Sodium: 43 mg.
- Protein: 2.3 g.
- Phosphorus: 198 mg.
- Potassium: 529 mg.

92. Grapes Jicama Salad

PREPARATION TIME

5'

COOK TIME

0'

SERVING

2

INGREDIENTS

- 1 jicama, peeled and sliced
- 1 carrot, sliced
- 1/2 medium red onion, sliced
- 1 1/4 cup grapes, seedless
- 1/3 cup fresh basil leaves
- 1 tbsp. apple cider vinegar
- 1 1/2 tbsp. lemon juice
- 1 1/2 tbsp. lime juice

DIRECTIONS

1. Put all the salad ingredients into a suitable salad bowl.
2. Toss them well and refrigerate for 1 hour.
3. Serve!

NUTRIENTS PER SERVING

- Calories: 203
- Protein: 3.7 g.
- Fat: 0.7 g.
- Sodium: 44 mg.
- Potassium: 429 mg.
- Phosphorus: 141 mg.

93. Cucumber Couscous Salad

PREPARATION TIME
5'

COOK TIME
0'

SERVING
4

INGREDIENTS

- 1 cucumber, sliced
- 1/2 cup red bell pepper, sliced
- 1/4 cup sweet onion, sliced
- 2 tbsp. black olives, sliced
- 1/4 cup parsley, chopped
- 1/2 cup couscous, cooked
- 2 tbsp. olive oil
- 2 tbsp. rice vinegar
- 2 tbsp. feta cheese, crumbled
- 1 1/2 tsp. dried basil
- 1/4 tsp. black pepper

DIRECTIONS

1. Put all the salad ingredients into a suitable salad bowl.
2. Toss them well and refrigerate for 1 hour.
3. Serve!

NUTRIENTS PER SERVING

- Calories: 202
- Protein: 6.2 g.
- Fat: 9.8 g.
- Sodium: 258 mg.
- Potassium: 209 mg.
- Phosphorus: 192 mg.

94. Carrot Jicama Salad

PREPARATION TIME
5'

COOK TIME
0'

SERVING
2

INGREDIENTS

- 2 cup carrots, julienned
- 1 1/2 cups jicama, julienned
- 2 tbsp. lime juice
- 1 tbsp. olive oil
- 1/2 tbsp. apple cider
- 1/2 tsp. brown Swerve

DIRECTIONS

1. Put all the salad ingredients into a suitable salad bowl.
2. Toss them well and refrigerate for 1 hour.
3. Serve!

NUTRIENTS PER SERVING

- Calories: 173
- Protein: 1.6 g.
- Fat: 7.1 g.
- Sodium: 80 mg.
- Potassium: 501 mg.
- Phosphorus: 96 mg.

95. Butterscotch Apple Salad

PREPARATION TIME
5'

COOK TIME
0'

SERVING
6

INGREDIENTS

- 3 cups jazz apples, chopped
- 8 oz. canned pineapple, crushed
- 8 oz. whipped topping
- 1/2 cup butterscotch topping
- 1/3 cup almonds
- 1/4 cup butterscotch chips
- 1/4 tsp. black pepper

DIRECTIONS

1. Put all the salad ingredients into a suitable salad bowl.
2. Toss them well and refrigerate for 1 hour.
3. Serve.

NUTRIENTS PER SERVING

- Calories: 293
- Protein: 4.2 g.
- Fat: 12.7 g.
- Sodium: 52 mg.
- Potassium: 296 mg.
- Phosphorus: 202 mg.

96. Cranberry Cabbage Slaw

PREPARATION TIME
10'

COOK TIME
0'

SERVING
4

INGREDIENTS

- 1/2 medium cabbage head, shredded
- 1 medium red apple, shredded
- 2 tbsp. onion, sliced
- 1/2 cup dried cranberries
- 1/4 cup almonds, toasted sliced
- 1/2 cup olive oil
- 1/4 tsp. stevia
- 1/4 cup cider vinegar
- 1/2 tbsp. celery seed
- 1/2 tsp. dry mustard
- 1/2 cup cream

DIRECTIONS

1. Take a suitable salad bowl.
2. Start tossing in all the ingredients.
3. Mix well and serve.

NUTRIENTS PER SERVING

- Calories: 308 g.
- Protein: 2.6 g.
- Fat: 24.5 g.
- Sodium: 23 mg.
- Potassium: 219 mg.
- Phosphorus: 257 mg.

97. Chestnut Noodle Salad

PREPARATION TIME
5'

COOK TIME
0'

SERVING
6

INGREDIENTS

- 8 cups cabbage, shredded
- 1/2 cup canned chestnuts, sliced
- 6 green onions, chopped
- 1/4 cup olive oil
- 1/4 cup apple cider vinegar
- 3/4 tsp. stevia
- 1/8 tsp. black pepper
- 1 cup Chow Mein noodles, cooked

DIRECTIONS

1. Take a suitable salad bowl.
2. Start tossing in all the ingredients.
3. Mix well and serve.

NUTRIENTS PER SERVING

- Calories: 191
- Protein: 4.2 g.
- Fat: 13 g.
- Sodium: 78 mg.
- Potassium: 302 mg.
- Phosphorus: 188 mg.

CHAPTER 18

Soups and Stews

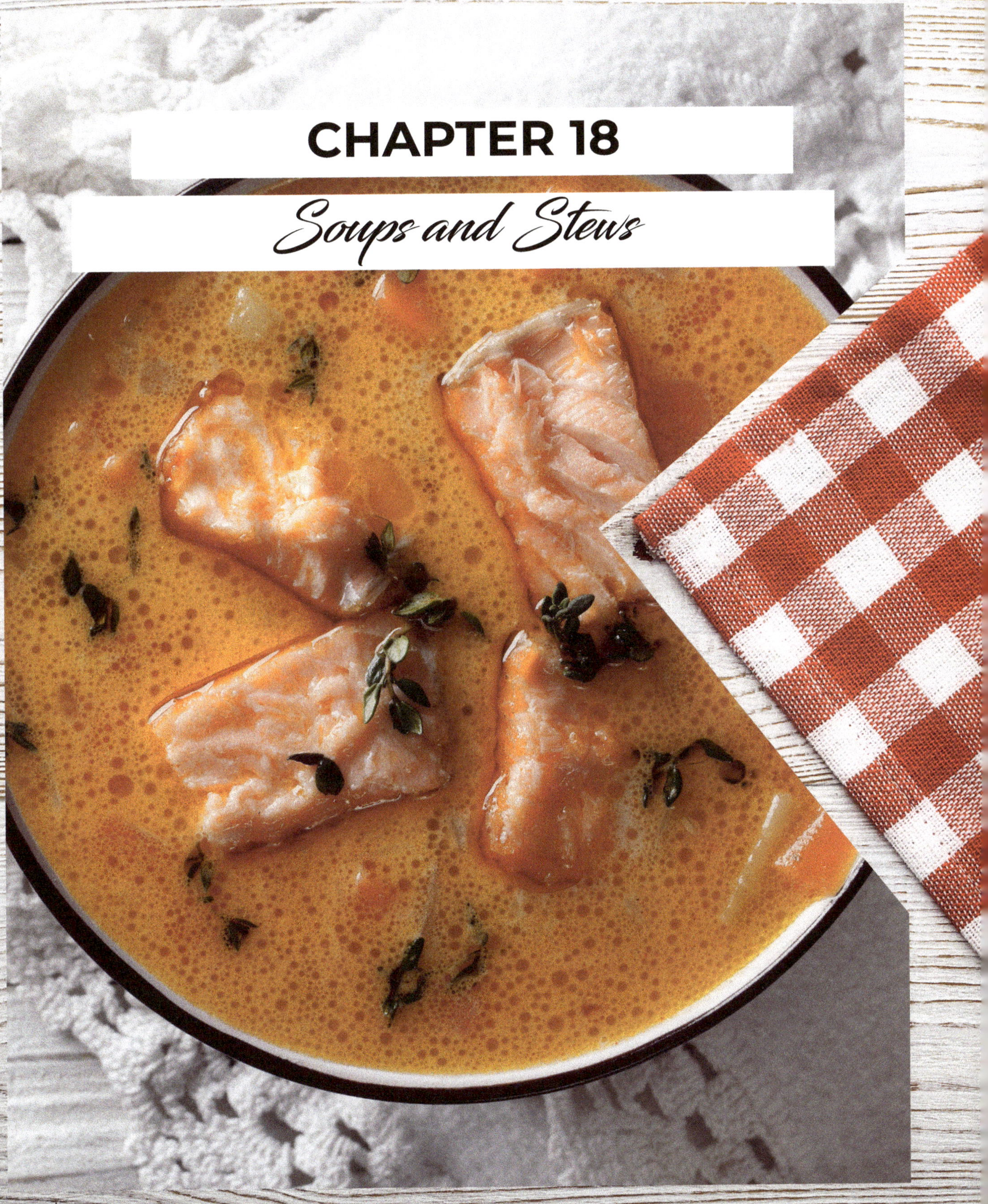

98. Yucatan Soup

PREPARATION TIME
10'

COOK TIME
20'

SERVING
4

INGREDIENTS

- 1/2 cup onion, chopped
- 8 cloves garlic, chopped
- 2 Serrano chili peppers, chopped
- 1 medium tomato, chopped
- 1 1/2 cups chicken breast, cooked, shredded
- 26-inch corn tortillas, sliced
- Nonstick cooking spray
- 1 tbsp. olive oil
- 4 cups chicken broth
- 1 bay leaf
- 1/4 cup lime juice
- 1/4 cup cilantro, chopped
- 1 tsp. black pepper

DIRECTIONS

1. Spread the corn tortillas on a baking sheet and bake them for 3 minutes at 400°F.
2. Place a suitably-sized saucepan over medium heat and add oil to heat.
3. Toss in chili peppers, garlic, and onion, then sauté until soft.
4. Stir in broth, tomatoes, bay leaf, and chicken.
5. Let this chicken soup cook for 10 minutes on a simmer.
6. Stir in cilantro, lime juice, and black pepper.
7. Garnish with baked corn tortillas.

NUTRIENTS PER SERVING

- Calories: 214
- Protein: 20 g.
- Fat: 10 g.
- Carb: 12 g.
- Sodium: 246 mg.
- Potassium: 355 mg.
- Phosphorus: 176 mg.

99. Zesty Taco Soup

PREPARATION TIME
10'

COOK TIME
7 HOURS

SERVING
2

INGREDIENTS

- 1/2 lb. boneless skinless chicken breast
- 15 canned dark red kidney beans (1/2 oz.)
- 15 canned white corn (1/2 oz.)
- 1 cup canned tomatoes, diced
- 1/2 cup onion
- 15 canned yellow hominy (1/2 oz.)
- 1/2 cup green bell peppers
- 1 garlic clove
- 1 medium jalapeño
- 1 tbsp. Package McCormick®
- 2 cups chicken broth

DIRECTIONS

1. Add drained beans, hominy, corn, onion, garlic, jalapeño pepper, chicken, and green peppers to a Crockpot.
2. Cover the beans-corn mixture and cook for 1 hour at high temperature.
3. Reduce the heat to low and continue cooking for 6 hours.
4. Shred the slow-cooked chicken and return to the taco soup.
5. Serve warm.

NUTRIENTS PER SERVING

- Calories: 210
- Protein: 21 g.
- Fat: 3 g.
- Carb: 19 g.
- Sodium: 421 mg.
- Potassium: 444 mg.
- Phosphorus: 210 mg.

100. Southwestern Posole

PREPARATION TIME
10'

COOK TIME
35'

SERVING
4

INGREDIENTS

- 1 lb. pork loin, diced
- 1 tbsp. olive oil
- 1/2 cup onion, chopped
- 1 garlic clove, chopped
- 28 oz. canned white hominy
- 4 oz. canned diced green chilies
- 4 cups chicken broth
- 1/4 tsp. black pepper

DIRECTIONS

1. Place a suitably-sized cooking pot over medium heat and add oil to heat.
2. Toss in pork pieces and sauté for 4 minutes.
3. Stir in garlic and onion, then stir for 4 minutes, or until onion is soft.
4. Add the remaining ingredients, then cover the pork soup.
5. Cook for 45 minutes, or until the pork is tender.
6. Serve warm.

NUTRIENTS PER SERVING

- Calories: 286
- Protein: 26 g.
- Fat: 13 g.
- Carb: 15 g.
- Sodium: 399 mg.
- Potassium: 346 mg.
- Phosphorus: 182 mg.

101. Spring Vegetable Soup

PREPARATION TIME
10'

COOK TIME
45'

SERVING
4

INGREDIENTS

- 1 cup fresh green beans, chopped
- 3/4 cup celery, chopped
- 1/2 cup onion, chopped
- 1/2 cup carrots, chopped
- 1/2 cup mushrooms, chopped
- 1/2 cup frozen corn
- 1 medium Roma tomato, chopped
- 2 tbsp. olive oil
- 1/2 cup frozen corn
- 4 cups vegetable broth
- 1 tsp. dried oregano leaves
- 1 tsp. garlic powder

DIRECTIONS

1. Place a suitably-sized cooking pot over medium heat and add olive oil to heat.
2. Toss in onion and celery, then sauté until soft.
3. Stir in the corn and rest of the ingredients and cook the soup to boil.
4. Now reduce its heat to a simmer and cook for 45 minutes.
5. Serve warm.

NUTRIENTS PER SERVING

- Calories: 114
- Protein: 2 g.
- Fat: 6 g.
- Carb: 13 g.
- Sodium: 262 mg.
- Potassium: 400 mg.
- Phosphorus: 108 mg.

102. Seafood Corn Chowder

PREPARATION TIME

10'

COOK TIME

12'

SERVING

4

INGREDIENTS

- 1 tbsp. butter
- 1 cup onion, chopped
- 1/3 cup celery, chopped
- 1/2 cup green bell pepper, chopped
- 1/2 cup red bell pepper, chopped
- 1 tbsp. white flour
- 14 oz. chicken broth
- 2 cups cream
- 6 oz. evaporated milk
- 10 oz. surimi imitation crab chunks
- 2 cups frozen corn kernels
- 1/2 tsp. black pepper
- 1/2 tsp. paprika

DIRECTIONS

1. Place a suitably-sized saucepan over medium heat and add butter to melt.
2. Toss in onion, green and red peppers, and celery, then sauté for 5 minutes.
3. Stir in flour and whisk well for 2 minutes.
4. Pour in chicken broth and stir until it boils.
5. Add evaporated milk, corn, surimi crab, paprika, black pepper, and creamer.
6. Cook for 5 minutes, then serve warm.

NUTRIENTS PER SERVING

- Calories: 173
- Protein: 8 g.
- Fat: 7 g.
- Carb: 22 g.
- Sodium: 160 mg.
- Potassium: 285 mg.
- Phosphorus: 181 mg.

103. Beef Sage Soup

PREPARATION TIME

10'

COOK TIME

20'

SERVING

4

INGREDIENTS

- 1/2 lb. ground beef
- 1/2 tsp. ground sage
- 1/2 tsp. black pepper
- 1/2 tsp. dried basil
- 1/2 tsp. garlic powder
- 4 slices bread, cubed
- 2 tbsp. olive oil
- 1 tbsp. herb seasoning blend
- 2 garlic cloves, minced
- 3 cups chicken broth
- 1 1/2 cups water
- 4 tbsp. fresh parsley
- 2 tbsp. parmesan cheese, grated

DIRECTIONS

1. Preheat your oven to 375°F.
2. Mix beef with sage, basil, black pepper, and garlic powder in a bowl, then set it aside.
3. Toss the bread cubes with olive oil on a baking sheet and bake them for 8 minutes.
4. Meanwhile, sauté the beef mixture in a greased cooking pot until it is browned.
5. Stir in garlic and sauté for 2 minutes, then add parsley, water, and broth.
6. Cover the beef soup and cook for 10 minutes on a simmer.
7. Garnish the soup with parmesan cheese and baked bread.

NUTRIENTS PER SERVING

- Calories: 335
- Protein: 26 g.
- Fat: 19 g.
- Carb: 15 g.
- Sodium: 374 mg.
- Potassium: 392 mg.
- Phosphorus: 268 mg.

104. Cabbage Borscht

PREPARATION TIME

10'

COOK TIME

1 H 1/2

SERVING

6

INGREDIENTS

- 2 lbs. beef steaks
- 6 cups cold water
- 2 tbsp. olive oil
- 1/2 cup tomato sauce
- 1 medium cabbage, chopped
- 1 cup onion, diced
- 1 cup carrots, diced
- 1 cup turnips, peeled and diced
- 1 tsp. pepper
- 6 tbsp. lemon juice
- 4 tbsp. sugar

DIRECTIONS

1. Start by placing steak in a large cooking pot and pour enough water to cover it.
2. Cover the beef pot and cook it on a simmer until it is tender, then shred it using a fork.
3. Add olive oil, onion, tomato sauce, carrots, turnips, and shredded steak to the cooking liquid in the pot.
4. Stir in black pepper, sugar, and lemon juice to season the soup.
5. Cover the cabbage soup and cook on low heat for 1 1/2 hour.

NUTRIENTS PER SERVING

- Calories: 202
- Protein: 19 g.
- Fat: 10 g.
- Carb: 9 g.
- Sodium: 242 mg.
- Potassium: 388 mg.
- Phosphorus: 160 mg.

105. Ground Beef Soup

PREPARATION TIME
10'

COOK TIME
30'

SERVING
4

INGREDIENTS

- 1 lb. lean ground beef
- 1/2 cup onion, chopped
- 2 tsp. lemon-pepper seasoning blend
- 1 cup beef broth
- 2 cups of water
- 1/3 cup white rice, uncooked
- 3 cups of frozen mixed vegetables
- 1 tbsp. sour cream

DIRECTIONS

1. Spray a saucepan with cooking oil and place it over medium heat.
2. Toss in onion and ground beef, then sauté until brown.
3. Stir in broth and rest of the ingredients, then boil it.
4. Reduce heat to a simmer, then cover the soup to cook for 30 minutes.
5. Garnish with sour cream.

NUTRIENTS PER SERVING

- Calories: 222
- Protein: 20 g.
- Fat: 8 g.
- Carb: 19 g.
- Sodium: 170 mg.
- Potassium: 448 mg.
- Phosphorus: 210 mg.

106. Shrimp and Crab Gumbo

PREPARATION TIME
10'

COOK TIME
15'

SERVING
4

INGREDIENTS

- 1 cup bell pepper, chopped
- 1 1/2 cups onion, chopped
- 1 garlic clove, chopped
- 1/4 cup celery leaves, chopped
- 1 cup green onion tops
- 1/4 cup fresh parsley, chopped
- 4 tbsp. canola oil
- 6 tbsp. all-purpose white flour
- 3 cups of water
- 4 cups chicken broth
- 8 oz. shrimp, uncooked
- 6 oz. crab meat
- 1/4 tsp. black pepper
- 1 tsp. hot sauce
- 3 cups cooked rice

DIRECTIONS

1. Prepare the roux in a suitably-sized pan by heating oil in it.
2. Stir in flour and sauté until it changes its color.
3. Pour in 1 cup water, then add onion, garlic, celery leaves, and bell pepper.
4. Cover the roux mixture and cook on low heat until the veggies turn soft.
5. Add 2 cups water and 4 cups broth, then mix again.
6. Continue cooking it for 5 minutes then add crab meat and shrimp.
7. Cook for 10 minutes then add parsley and green onion.
8. Continue cooking for 5 minutes then garnish with black pepper and hot sauce.
9. Serve warm with rice.

NUTRIENTS PER SERVING

- Calories: 327
- Protein: 22 g.
- Fat: 11 g.
- Carb: 33 g.
- Sodium: 328 mg.
- Potassium: 368 mg.
- Phosphorus: 221 mg.

107. Tangy Turkey Soup

PREPARATION TIME
10'

COOK TIME
68'

SERVING
4

INGREDIENTS

- 1 cup carrots, chopped
- 1 cup celery, chopped
- 1 cup green bell pepper, chopped
- 1 cup yellow onion, chopped
- 1/2 cup fresh tomato, chopped
- 1/2 cup fresh parsley, chopped
- 2 garlic cloves, chopped
- 1 cup mushrooms, sliced
- 2 cups zucchini, sliced
- 1 tbsp. olive oil
- 1 lb. turkey breast, skinless, cubed
- 1/2 tsp. black pepper
- 1/2 cup dry white wine
- 4 cups chicken broth
- 1 tsp. dried thyme
- 1 bay leaf
- 1/4 tsp. crushed red pepper
- 3 cups white rice, cooked
- 3 tbsp. lemon juice

DIRECTIONS

1. Place a suitably-sized stockpot over medium heat and oil to heat.
2. Toss in turkey, and black pepper, then sauté for 10 minutes.
3. Stir in green bell pepper, onion, celery, and carrots, then sauté for 8 minutes.
4. Add garlic, tomato, and wine then cook for 2 minutes.
5. Stir in bay leaf, thyme, broth, and red pepper then cook for 30 minutes on a simmer.
6. Add zucchini, mushrooms, parsley, and rice to the soup then continue cooking for 15 minutes.
7. Serve warm with lemon juice on top.

NUTRIENTS PER SERVING

- Calories: 214
- Protein: 18 g.
- Fat: 6 g.
- Carb: 22 g.
- Sodium: 128 mg.
- Potassium: 528 mg.
- Phosphorus: 197 mg.

108. Chicken Soup

PREPARATION TIME
20'

COOK TIME
30'

SERVING
8

INGREDIENTS

- 1 lb. chicken breast, boneless, skinless
- 1 cup yellow onion, chopped
- 1 cup celery, chopped
- 1 cup sliced carrots
- 1 cup fresh beans cut into 2-inch pieces
- 1 cup green peas
- 1/4 tsp. nutmeg
- 1 tsp. thyme
- 1 tsp. oregano
- 32 oz. reduced-sodium chicken broth
- 1/2 cup low-fat milk (1%)
- 1/4 tsp. black pepper
- 3 tbsp. white floor
- 1 tbsp. olive oil
- 3 cup of water

DIRECTIONS

1. First, cook and shred chicken by coating the bottom of a deep-frying pan with olive oil on medium heat for 5 minutes. Remove from heat.
2. Then place the chicken in a pan and cook for 5 minutes. Flip to the other side and add 3/4 cup of water.
3. In a separate large skillet sauté onion, carrots, and celery for 4–5 minutes.
4. Add chicken and all other ingredients (beans, peas, flour, oregano, thyme, and nutmeg) and cook on medium. Mix and cook for 5 minutes.
5. Add broth and milk, boil for 5 minutes.
6. Add pepper to taste.

NUTRIENTS PER SERVING

- Calories: 133
- Protein: 15 g.
- Fat: 3 g.
- Carb: 13 g.
- Sodium: 343 mg.
- Potassium: 465 mg.
- Phosphorus: 101 mg.

109. Curried Onion and Cauliflower Soup

PREPARATION TIME
10'

COOK TIME
40'

SERVING
4

INGREDIENTS

- 2 tbsp. coconut oil
- 1 onion, peeled and chopped
- 4 cloves garlic, minced
- 1/2 cauliflower, chopped
- 3 sliced celeries, chopped
- 1 tsp. cumin
- 1 tsp. turmeric
- 1 cup homemade chicken stock
- 3 cups of water
- 1 cup low fat coconut milk

DIRECTIONS

1. Heat the oil in a large pan over medium to high heat.
2. Add the onions, garlic, and cauliflower and sweat for 5–10 minutes (don't let them brown).
3. Add the celery and spices and cook for another 5 minutes.
4. Add the stock and water and bring to a boil before lowering the heat and simmering for 15–20 minutes or until celery is soft.
5. Remove from heat and allow to cool before blending in a food processor or liquidizer (don't panic if you don't have one, you can enjoy this soup as a chunky soup!)
6. Return to the pan and add the coconut milk, warming through.
7. Serve with a sprinkle of black pepper.

Tip: Check with your doctor or dietitian as to whether you can still have coconut milk. Alternatively use non-dairy milk such as almond.

NUTRIENTS PER SERVING

- Calories: 184
- Protein: 4 g.
- Fat: 15 g.
- Carb: 13 g.
- Sodium: 59 mg.
- Potassium: 400 mg.
- Phosphorus: 94 mg.

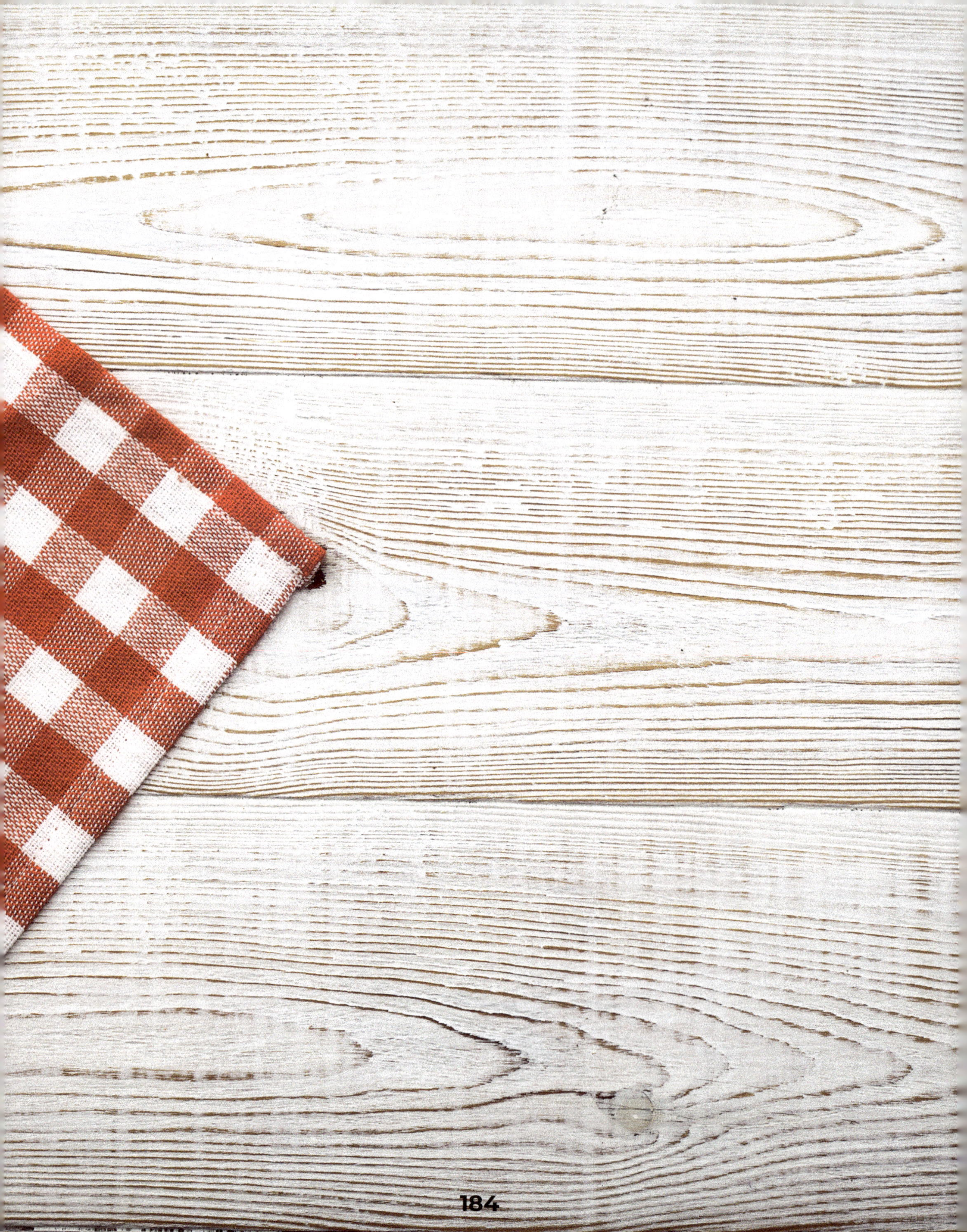

CHAPTER 19

Sauces, Condiments and Seasoning Blends

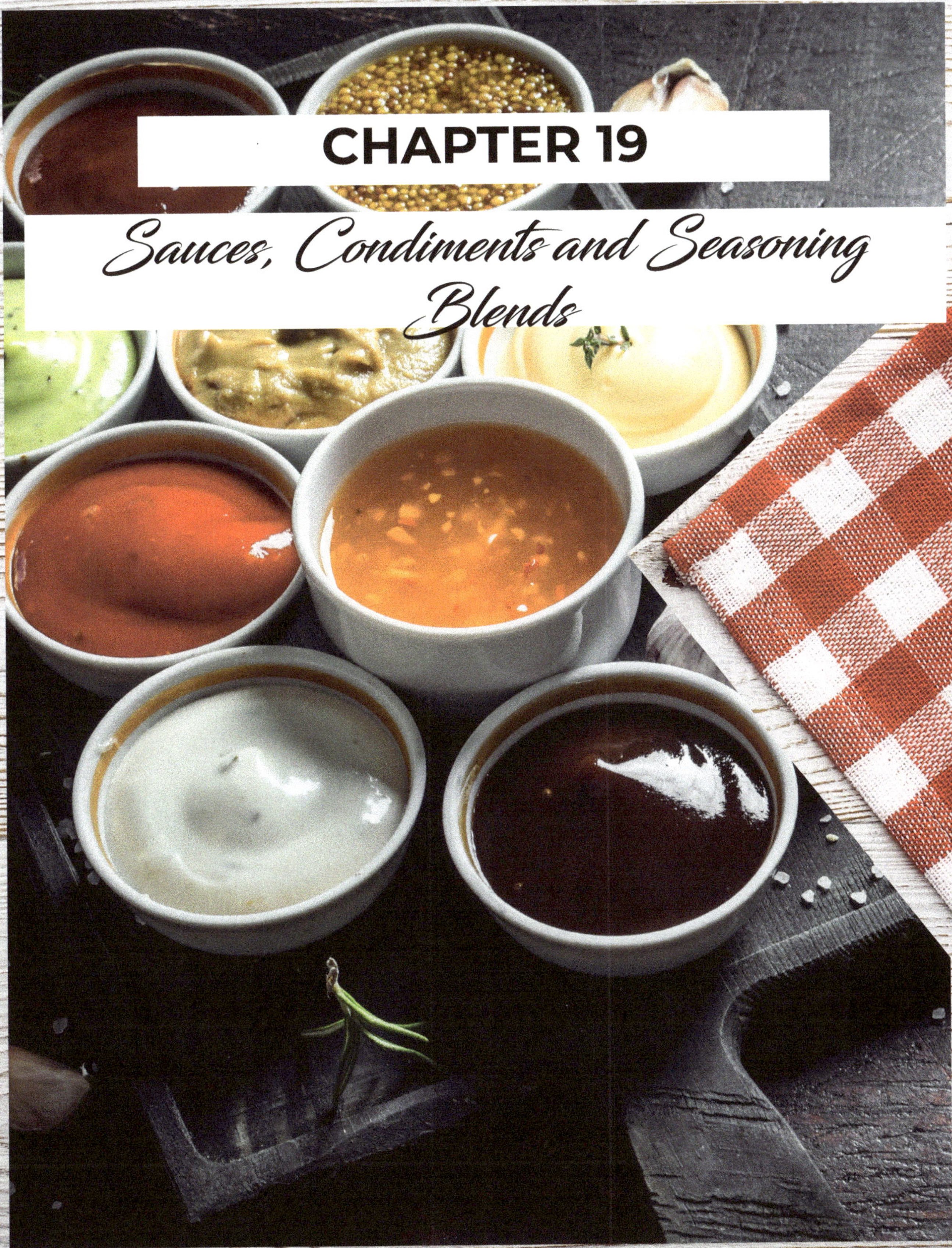

110. Easy Garlicky Cherry Tomato Sauce

PREPARATION TIME

5'

COOK TIME

25'

SERVING

5

INGREDIENTS

- 1/4 cup extra virgin olive oil
- 1/4 garlic cloves, thinly sliced
- 2 lb. organic cherry tomatoes
- 1/2 tsp. dried oregano
- 1 tsp. coconut sugar
- 1/4 cup fresh basil, chopped
- 1 tsp. salt

DIRECTIONS

1. Heat oil in a large pot over average heat.
2. Sauté the garlic for a minute until fragrant.
3. Add in the cherry tomatoes and season with salt, oregano, coconut sugar, and fresh basil.
4. Allow simmering for 25 minutes until the tomatoes are soft and become a thick sauce.
5. Place in containers and store in the fridge until ready to use.

NUTRIENTS PER SERVING

- Calories: 198
- Protein: 3 g.
- Sodium: 116 mg.
- Potassium: 514 mg.
- Phosphorus: 316 mg.

111. Avocado Cilantro Detox Dressing

PREPARATION TIME
5'

COOK TIME
0'

SERVING
5

INGREDIENTS

- 5 tbsp. lemon juice, freshly squeezed
- 1 clove of garlic, chopped
- 1 avocado, pitted and flesh scooped out
- 1 bunch cilantro, chopped
- 1/4 tsp. salt
- 1/4 cup water

DIRECTIONS

1. In a food processor, place all ingredients and pulse until well combined.
2. Pulse until creamy.
3. Place in a lidded container and store in the fridge until ready to use.
4. Use on salads and sandwiches.

NUTRIENTS PER SERVING

- Calories: 114
- Protein: 2 g.
- Sodium: 5 mg.
- Potassium: 355 mg.
- Phosphorus: 256 mg.

112. Golden Turmeric Sauce

PREPARATION TIME
10'

COOK TIME
15'

SERVING
4

INGREDIENTS

- 2 tbsp. coconut oil
- 1 onion, chopped
- 2-inch piece ginger, peeled and minced
- 2 cloves of garlic, minced
- 2 cups white sweet potato, cubed
- 2 tbsp. turmeric powder
- 1/2 tsp. ginger powder
- 1/4 tsp. cinnamon powder
- 2 cups of coconut milk
- Juice from 1 lemon, freshly squeezed
- 1 cup of water
- 1 1/2 tsp. salt

DIRECTIONS

1. In a saucepan, heat oil at medium heat.
2. Sauté the onion, ginger, and garlic until fragrant.
3. Add in the sweet potatoes, turmeric powder, ginger powder, and cinnamon powder.
4. Pour in water and season with salt.
5. Bring to a boil for 10 minutes.
6. Once the potatoes are soft, place in a blender and pulse until smooth.
7. Return the mixture into the saucepan. Turn on the stove.
8. Add in the coconut milk and lemon juice.
9. Allow simmering for 5 minutes.
10. Store in lidded containers and put inside the fridge until ready to use.

NUTRIENTS PER SERVING

- Calories: 172
- Protein: 5 g.
- Sodium: 36 mg.
- Potassium: 408 mg.
- Phosphorus: 216 mg.

113. Creamy Turmeric Dressing

PREPARATION TIME
5'

COOK TIME
0'

SERVING
6

INGREDIENTS

- 1/2 cup tahini
- 1/2 cup olive oil
- 2 tbsp. lemon juice
- 2 tsp. honey
- Salt to taste
- A dash of black pepper

DIRECTIONS

1. Mix all ingredients in a bowl until the mixture becomes creamy and smooth.
2. Store in lidded containers.
3. Put in the fridge until ready to use.

NUTRIENTS PER SERVING

- Calories: 286
- Protein: 4 g.
- Sodium: 24 mg.
- Potassium: 89 mg.
- Phosphorus: 316 mg.

114. Dijon Mustard Vinaigrette

PREPARATION TIME
5'

COOK TIME
0'

SERVING
6

INGREDIENTS

- 3/4 cup olive oil
- 1/4 cup apple cider vinegar
- 3 tbsp. Dijon mustard
- 2 shallots, quartered
- 1 garlic clove, chopped
- A handful of parsley, chopped

DIRECTIONS

1. Place all ingredients in a food processor.
2. Pulse until smooth.
3. Place in containers and store in the fridge until ready to use.

NUTRIENTS PER SERVING

- Calories: 252
- Protein: 0.6 g.
- Sodium: 80 mg.
- Potassium: 93 mg.
- Phosphorous 146 mg.

115. Low Phosphorus Baking Powder

PREPARATION TIME
10'

COOK TIME
20'

SERVING
8

INGREDIENTS

- 6 tbsp. cream of tartar
- 3 tbsp. baking soda
- 1 tbsp. cornstarch

DIRECTIONS

1. Add the cream of tartar, cornstarch, and baking powder in a small bowl and whisk to combine.
2. Force the mixture through a fine sieve to remove any lumps.
3. Pile in an airtight bowl at room temperature and use in baking recipes.

NUTRIENTS PER SERVING

- Calories: 6
- Protein: 0 g.
- Fat: 2 g.
- Carb: 1 g.
- Sodium: 379 mg.
- Potassium: 297 mg.
- Phosphorus: 0 mg.

116. Every Day No-Salt Seasoning Blend

PREPARATION TIME
10'

COOK TIME
2'

SERVING
2

INGREDIENTS

- 1 tsp. dried thyme leaves
- 1 tsp. dried marjoram leaves
- 1 tsp. dried basil leaves
- 1 tsp. dried oregano leaves
- 1/2 tsp. onion powder
- 1/2 tsp. garlic powder
- 1/2 tsp. ground mustard
- 1/4 tsp. freshly ground black pepper
- 1/4 tsp. paprika

DIRECTIONS

1. Combine the thyme, marjoram, basil, oregano, onion powder, garlic powder, ground mustard, pepper, and paprika furthermore, keep in a little container with a tight cover at room temperature for up to 6 months.

NUTRIENTS PER SERVING

- Calories: 4
- Protein: 0 g.
- Fat: 0 g.
- Carb: 1 g.
- Sodium: 1 mg.
- Potassium: 17 mg.
- Phosphorus: 4 mg

117. Thai-Style Seasoning Blend

PREPARATION TIME
10'

COOK TIME
2'

SERVING
3

INGREDIENTS

- 1 1/2 tsp. turmeric
- 11/2 tsp. paprika
- 1 tsp. ground coriander
- 1 tsp. ground ginger
- 1 tsp. dry mustard
- 1 tsp. ground cumin
- 1 tsp. dried mint leaves, crushed
- 1 tsp. red pepper flakes

DIRECTIONS

1. Combine the turmeric, paprika, coriander, ginger, dry mustard, cumin, mint, and red pepper flakes and keep in a small jar with a tight lid at room temperature for up to 6 months.

NUTRIENTS PER SERVING

- Calories: 5
- Protein: 0 g.
- Fat: 0 g.
- Carb: 1 g.
- Sodium: 1 mg.
- Potassium: 30 mg.
- Phosphorus: 6 mg.

118. Tex-Mex Seasoning Mix

PREPARATION TIME
10'

COOK TIME
2'

SERVING
2

INGREDIENTS

- 1 tbsp. chili powder
- 1/2 tsp. ground cumin
- 1/2 tsp. dried oregano leaves
- 1/2 tsp. garlic powder
- 1/2 tsp. onion powder
- 1/2 tsp. cayenne pepper
- 1/2 tsp. red pepper flakes

DIRECTIONS

1. Combine the chili powder, cumin, oregano, garlic powder, onion powder, cayenne pepper, and red pepper drops and keep in a little container with a tight top at room temperature for up to 6 months.

NUTRIENTS PER SERVING

- Calories: 7
- Protein: 0 g.
- Carb: 1 g.
- Fat: 0 g.
- Sodium: 39 mg.
- Potassium: 38 mg.
- Phosphorus: 7 mg.

119. Duxelles

PREPARATION TIME
15'

COOK TIME
15'

SERVING
8

INGREDIENTS

- 1 (8 oz.) cremini mushrooms, package sliced
- 3 scallions, white and green parts
- 3 garlic cloves
- 1 tbsp. olive oil
- 1 tbsp. unsalted butter
- 1 tsp. lemon juice, freshly squeezed
- Pinch salt

DIRECTIONS

1. Finely chop the mushrooms, scallions, and garlic in a food processor or blender.
2. Place the mushroom blend in the center of a kitchen towel, gather up the ends to create a pouch, and squeeze the pouch over the sink to remove some of the liquid in the mushrooms.
3. Heat the olive oil and butter in a large skillet over medium-high heat.
4. Add the drained mushroom mixture to the skillet and sprinkle with the lemon juice and salt.
5. Sauté for 8–12 minutes, stirring frequently, or until the mushrooms are browned.
6. This mixture can be refrigerated for up to 4 days or frozen for up to 1 month.

NUTRIENTS PER SERVING

- Calories: 37
- Protein: 1 g.
- Fat: 3 g.
- Carb: 2 g.
- Sodium: 22 mg.
- Potassium: 141 mg.
- Phosphorus: 37 mg.

120. Vegetable Broth

PREPARATION TIME
20'

COOK TIME
5'

SERVING
4

INGREDIENTS

- 1 tbsp. olive oil
- 1 onion, unpeeled, sliced
- 2 garlic cloves, unpeeled, crushed
- 2 carrots, unpeeled, sliced
- 2 celery stalks, cut into 2-inch pieces
- 1 bay leaf
- 1 tsp. dried basil leaves
- 5 cups of water

DIRECTIONS

1. In a big pot, warm olive oil over medium-high heat.
2. Sauté the onion, garlic, carrot, and celery for 5 minutes, stirring frequently, or until lightly browned.
3. Add the bay leaf, basil, and water to the saucepan and cook.
4. Decrease the temperature and cook for 20–22 minutes, stirring occasionally. Glide off and remove any scum that rises to the surface.
5. Strain the stock through a fine-mesh colander into a bowl. Discard the solids.
6. Refrigerate the broth and remove any fat that rises to the top. You can freeze this broth in 1-cup measures to use in recipes.
7. Stock in the freezer for up to 3 days; freeze for up to 3 months.

NUTRIENTS PER SERVING

- Calories: 31
- Protein: 0 g.
- Fat: 2 g.
- Carb: 4 g.
- Sodium: 21 mg.
- Potassium: 110 mg.
- Phosphorus: 14 mg.

CHAPTER 20

Eggs and Dairy

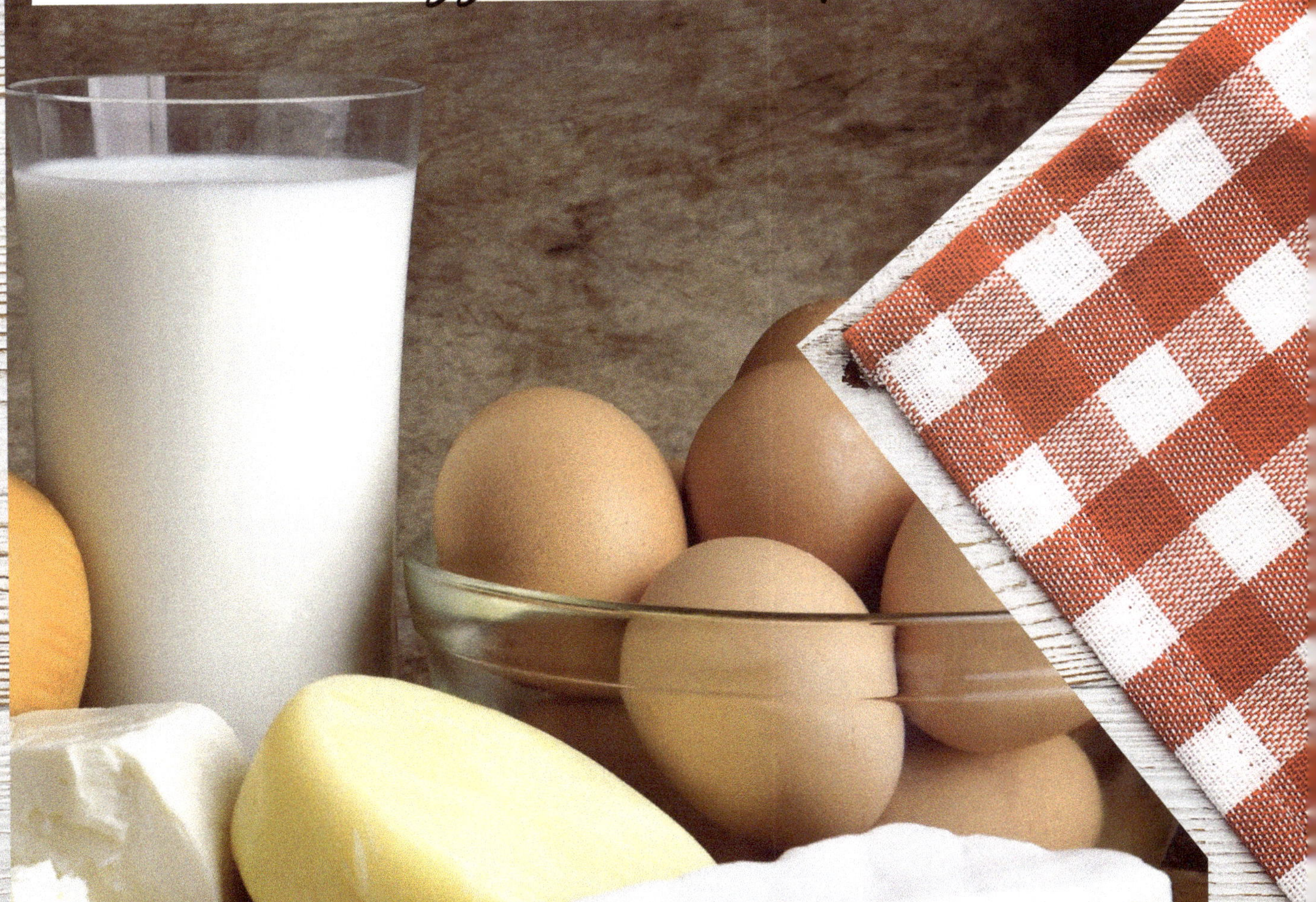

121. Cheese Stuffed Peppers

PREPARATION TIME
20'

COOK TIME
20'

SERVING
4

INGREDIENTS

- 4 summer bell peppers, cored and de-seeded
- 2 oz. mozzarella cheese, crumbled
- 2 tbsp. Greek yogurt
- 4 oz. cream cheese
- 1 clove garlic, minced

DIRECTIONS

1. Boil the peppers until they are just tender.
2. Thoroughly combine the cheese, yogurt, and garlic. Stuff your peppers with this filling. Place the stuffed peppers in a foil-lined baking dish.
3. Bake in the preheated oven at 365°F for about 10 minutes. Bon appétit!

NUTRIENTS PER SERVING

- Calories: 140
- Protein: 7 g.
- Fat: 9 g.
- Carb: 6 g.
- Sodium: 129 mg.
- Potassium: 227 mg.
- Phosphorus: 316 mg.

122. Italian Zucchini Sandwiches

PREPARATION TIME
25'

COOK TIME
0'

SERVING
4

INGREDIENTS

- 4 thin zucchini slices, cut lengthwise
- 2 eggs
- 4 slices Sopressata
- 2 slices provolone cheese
- 1 red bell pepper, sliced thinly

DIRECTIONS

1. Dissolve 1 tbsp. of butter in a frying pan over medium-high flame. Then, fry the eggs for about 5 minutes.
2. Place one zucchini slice on each plate. Add the cheese, Sopressata, and peppers on top; season with salt and black pepper to taste.
3. Add fried eggs and top with the remaining zucchini slices. Bon appétit!

NUTRIENTS PER SERVING

- Calories: 240
- Protein: 7 g.
- Fat: 9 g.
- Carb: 6 g.
- Sodium: 131 mg.
- Potassium: 127 mg.
- Phosphorus: 216 mg.

123. Creamy Dilled Egg Salad

PREPARATION TIME
20'

COOK TIME
0'

SERVING
4

INGREDIENTS

- 2 eggs, peeled and chopped
- 1 scallion, chopped
- 1 tbsp. fresh dill minced
- 1 tsp. Dijon mustard
- 2 tbsp. mayonnaise

DIRECTIONS

1. Add the eggs and water to a saucepan and bring to a boil; remove from heat. Allow the eggs to sit, covered, for about 11 minutes.
2. Peel and rinse the eggs under running water. Then, chop the eggs and transfer them to a nice salad bowl; stir in the scallions, dill, mustard, and mayonnaise.
3. Taste and season with salt and pepper. Enjoy!

NUTRIENTS PER SERVING

- Calories: 220
- Protein: 5 g.
- Fat: 7 g.
- Carb: 6 g.
- Sodium: 142 mg.
- Potassium: 227 mg.
- Phosphorus: 316 mg.

124. Eggs With Goat Cheese

PREPARATION TIME
10'

COOK TIME
0'

SERVING
2

INGREDIENTS

- 4 eggs, whisked
- 2 tsp. ghee, room temperature
- 1 tsp. paprika
- Sea salt and ground black pepper, to taste
- 4 tbsp. goat cheese

DIRECTIONS

1. In a frying pan, melt the ghee over medium heat. Then, cook the eggs, covered, for about 4 minutes.
2. Stir in goat cheese, paprika, salt, and black pepper; continue to cook for 2–3 minutes more or until cooked through.
3. Taste and adjust seasonings. Enjoy!

NUTRIENTS PER SERVING

- Calories: 210
- Protein: 7 g.
- Fat: 9 g.
- Carb: 4 g.
- Sodium: 123 mg.
- Potassium: 227 mg.
- Phosphorus: 206 mg.

125. Dukkah Frittata With Cheese

PREPARATION TIME
30'

COOK TIME
0'

SERVING
2

INGREDIENTS

- 2 tbsp. low-fat milk
- 1 tbsp. Dukkah spice mix
- 3 eggs
- 1 1/2 tbsp. olive oil
- 1 cup cheddar cheese, shredded

DIRECTIONS

1. Preheat your oven to 360°F.
2. Whisk the milk, spices mix, and eggs until well mixed.
3. Grease the bottom of a small-sized baking pan with olive oil. Spoon the egg mixture into the pan and top with cheese.
4. Bake in the preheated oven for about 25 minutes until the eggs are set but the center jiggles just a bit. Bon appétit!

NUTRIENTS PER SERVING

- Calories: 330
- Protein: 11 g.
- Fat: 13 g.
- Carb: 6 g.
- Sodium: 119 mg.
- Potassium: 231 mg.
- Phosphorus: 319 mg.

126. Classic Italian Omelet

PREPARATION TIME
15'

COOK TIME
0'

SERVING
3

INGREDIENTS

- 6 oz. bacon, diced
- 2 Italian pepper, chopped
- 12 eggs, whisked
- 1 1/2 tsp. Italian seasoning blend
- 1 cup goat cheese, shredded

DIRECTIONS

1. Over medium-high heat, warm the frying pan. Now, fry the bacon until crisp or 3–4 minutes; set aside.
2. Stir in Italian pepper and continue to sauté for 2 minutes more, or until just tender and fragrant. Pour the eggs into the pan.
3. Sprinkle with the Italian seasoning blend; add the salt and black pepper to taste and cook until the eggs are set. Top with the reserved bacon and goat cheese.
4. Slide your omelet onto serving plates and serve. Bon appétit!

NUTRIENTS PER SERVING

- Calories: 308
- Protein: 10 g.
- Fat: 12 g.
- Carb: 6 g.
- Sodium: 122 mg.
- Potassium: 147 mg.
- Phosphorus: 126 mg.

127. Egg Salad With Anchovies

PREPARATION TIME

15'

COOK TIME

0'

SERVING

3

INGREDIENTS

- 3 oz. anchovies, flaked
- 5 eggs
- 2 tbsp. mayonnaise
- 1 tsp. Dijon mustard
- 2 tbsp. ricotta cheese

DIRECTIONS

1. Add the eggs and water to a pot and heat to the point of boiling; eliminate from heat. Permit the eggs to sit, secured, for around 11 minutes.
2. Then, peel the eggs and rinse them under running water. Then, transfer chopped eggs to a salad bowl.
3. Add in the remaining ingredients, gently stir to combine, and enjoy!

NUTRIENTS PER SERVING

- Calories: 240
- Protein: 7 g.
- Fat: 9 g.
- Carb: 6 g.
- Protein: 7 g.
- Sodium: 129 mg.
- Potassium: 227 mg.
- Phosphorus: 316 mg.

128. Classic Keto Cheesy Muffins With Almond Flour

PREPARATION TIME
10'

COOK TIME
35'

SERVING
4

INGREDIENTS

- 4 oz. cheddar cheese, shredded
- 6 tbsp. almond flour
- 2 tbsp. flaxseed meal
- 4 eggs
- 1/4 tsp. baking soda

DIRECTIONS

1. Start by preheating an oven at 355°F
2. Thoroughly combine all of the above ingredients until well mixed.
3. Coat a muffin pan with cupcake liners. Spoon the batter into the muffin pan. Bake in the preheated oven for 16 minutes.
4. Place on a wire rack for 10 minutes before unmolding and serving. Enjoy!

NUTRIENTS PER SERVING

- Calories: 213
- Protein: 7 g.
- Fat: 9 g.
- Sodium: 129 mg.
- Potassium: 209 mg.
- Phosphorus: 216 mg.

129. Authentic Spanish Migas

PREPARATION TIME
15

COOK TIME
10'

SERVING
3

INGREDIENTS

- 6 eggs
- 6 lettuce leaves
- 1 white onion, chopped
- 1 tomato, chopped
- 1 Spanish pepper, chopped

DIRECTIONS

1. Melt 1 tbsp. of butter in a cast-iron skillet over medium-high flame. Sauté the onion for about 4 minutes, stirring continuously to ensure even cooking.
2. Stir in the peppers and continue to sauté for an additional 3–4 minutes. Whisk in the eggs. Continue to cook until the eggs are set.
3. Divide the egg mixture between lettuce leaves; top with tomatoes. Season with salt and black pepper and serve. Devour!

NUTRIENTS PER SERVING

- Calories: 256
- Protein: 10 g.
- Fat: 8 g.
- Carb: 6 g.
- Sodium: 141 mg.
- Potassium: 127 mg.
- Phosphorus: 176 mg.

130. Double Cheese Fondue

PREPARATION TIME
10'

COOK TIME
0'

SERVING
8

INGREDIENTS

- 4 oz. ricotta cheese
- 1 cup double cream
- Cayenne pepper, to taste
- 8 oz. Swiss cheese, shredded
- 4 tbsp. Greek yogurt

DIRECTIONS

1. Warm Ricotta cheese and double cream and in a saucepan over a medium-low flame.
2. Remove from the heat. Fold in cayenne pepper, Swiss cheese, and Greek yogurt. Stir until everything is well combined.
3. Bon appétit!

NUTRIENTS PER SERVING

- Calories: 230
- Protein: 7 g.
- Fat: 9 g.
- Carb: 6 g.
- Sodium: 129 mg.
- Potassium: 209 mg.
- Phosphorus: 216 mg.

131. Savory Rolls With Bacon and Cheese

PREPARATION TIME
15-20'

COOK TIME
15'

SERVING
4

INGREDIENTS

- 1/4 cup goat cheese, crumbled
- 1/4 cup cream cheese
- 4 eggs
- 3 oz. bacon, diced
- 1/4 cup marinara sauce

DIRECTIONS

1. In a coated skillet, fry the bacon over the highest heat until crisp; set aside.
2. Whisk the cream cheese and eggs until foamy. Add in the fried bacon along with salt and black pepper; whisk to combine well.
3. Spoon the mixture into greased muffin cups. Top each muffin with goat cheese. Bake in the heated oven at 355°F for about 14 minutes or until golden on the top.
4. Serve with marinara sauce and enjoy!

NUTRIENTS PER SERVING

- Calories: 308
- Protein: 12 g.
- Fat: 9 g.
- Carb: 9 g.
- Sodium: 123 mg.
- Potassium: 217 mg.
- Phosphorus: 116 mg.

132. Broccoli Cheese Pie

PREPARATION TIME
5'

COOK TIME
30'

SERVING
4

INGREDIENTS

- 6 eggs
- 1 red onion, sliced
- 6 tbsp. Greek yogurt
- 2 cups broccoli florets
- 1/2 cup cheddar cheese, shredded

DIRECTIONS

1. Heat 2 tsp. of olive oil in an oven-safe skillet over medium-high heat. Sweat red onion and broccoli until they have softened or about 4 minutes.
2. Season with salt and black pepper.
3. In a mixing bowl, whisk Greek yogurt and eggs until well mixed. Scrape the mixture into the pan.
4. Bake at 365°F for 15–20 minutes or until a toothpick inserted into a muffin comes out dry and clean.
5. Top with cheddar cheese and bake for 5–6 minutes more. Bon appétit!

NUTRIENTS PER SERVING

- Calories: 140
- Protein: 7 g.
- Fat: 9 g.
- Carb: 6 g.
- Sodium: 129 mg.
- Potassium: 267 mg.
- Phosphorus: 316 mg.

CHAPTER 21

Vegetarian and Vegan

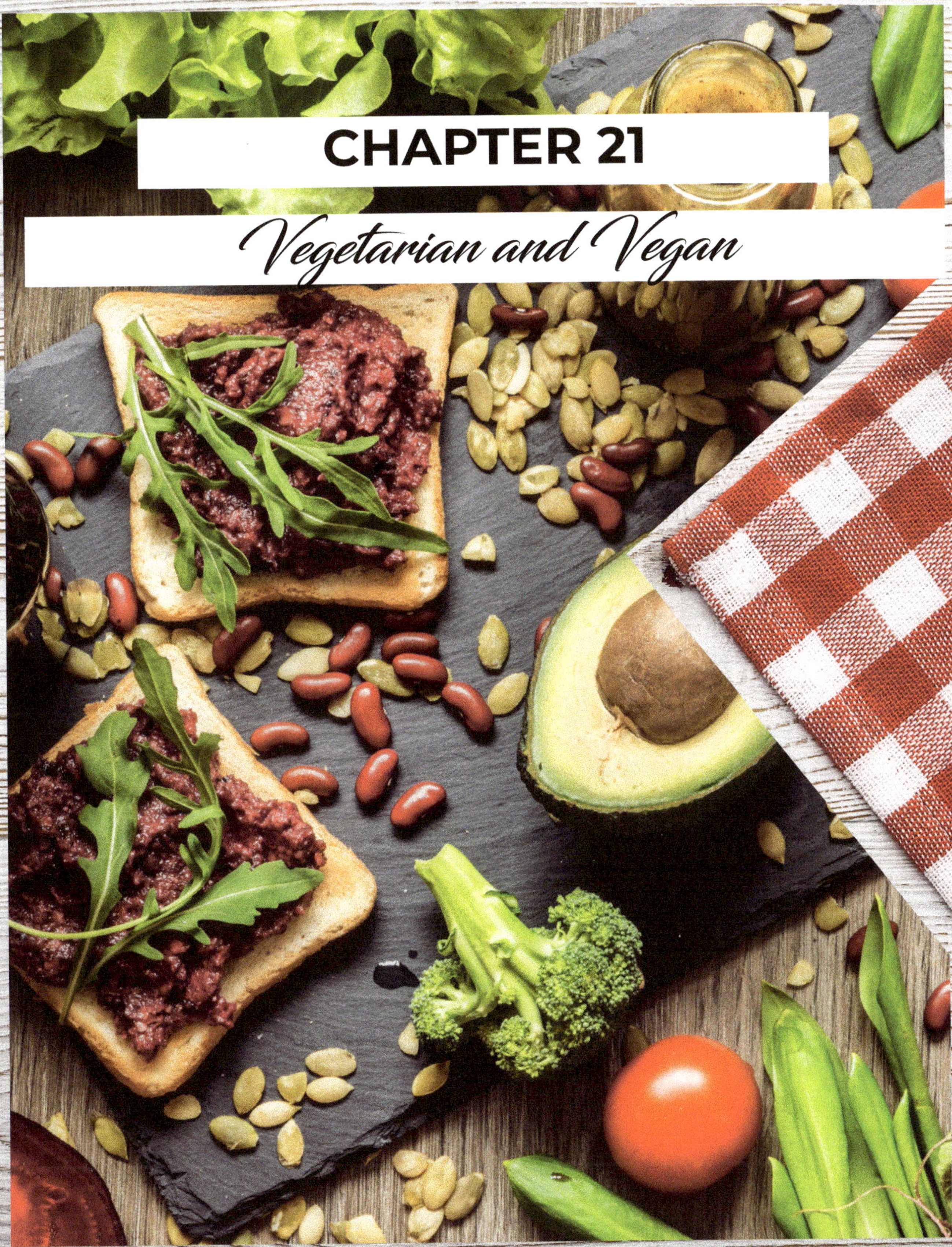

133. Curried Veggies and Rice

PREPARATION TIME
10'

COOK TIME
20'

SERVING
4

INGREDIENTS

- 1 cup long-grain white basmati rice
- 1/4 cup olive oil
- 4 garlic cloves, minced
- 2 1/2 tsp. curry powder
- 1/2 cup shiitake mushrooms, sliced
- 1 red bell pepper, chopped
- 1 cup frozen edamame, shelled
- 2 cups low-sodium vegetable broth
- 1/8 tsp. freshly ground black pepper

DIRECTIONS

1. Warm the olive oil over standard heat in a large pot.
2. Add the rice, garlic, curry powder, mushrooms, bell pepper, and edamame; cook, stirring, for 2 minutes.
3. Add the broth and black pepper and bring to a boil.
4. Reduce the heat to low, partially cover the pot, and simmer for 15–18 minutes or until the rice is tender. Stir and serve.

NUTRIENTS PER SERVING

- Calories: 347
- Protein: 8 g.
- Fat: 16 g.
- Carb: 44 g.
- Sodium: 114 mg.
- Potassium: 334 mg.
- Phosphorus: 131 mg.

134. Spicy Mushroom Stir-Fry

PREPARATION TIME
15'

COOK TIME
10'

SERVING
4

INGREDIENTS

- 2 (8 oz.) packages sliced button mushrooms
- 1 cup low-sodium vegetable broth
- 2 tbsp. cornstarch
- 1 tsp. low-sodium soy sauce
- 1/2 tsp. ground ginger
- 1/8 tsp. cayenne pepper
- 1 red bell pepper, chopped
- 1 jalapeño pepper, minced
- 3 cups brown rice that has been cooked in unsalted water
- 2 tbsp. sesame oil
- 2 tbsp. olive oil

DIRECTIONS

1. In a small bowl, whisk together the broth, cornstarch, soy sauce, ginger, and cayenne pepper and set aside.
2. Heat the olive oil in a wok or heavy skillet over high heat.
3. Add the mushrooms and peppers and stir-fry for 3–5 minutes or until the vegetables are tender-crisp.
4. Mix the broth combination and add it to the wok; stir-fry for 3–5 minutes longer or until the vegetables are tender and the sauce has thickened.
5. Serve the stir-fry over the hot cooked brown rice and drizzle with the sesame oil.

NUTRIENTS PER SERVING

- Calories: 361
- Protein: 8 g.
- Fat: 16 g.
- Carb: 49 g.
- Sodium: 95 mg.
- Potassium: 582 mg.
- Phosphorus: 267 mg.

135. Spicy Veggie Pancakes

PREPARATION TIME
20'

COOK TIME
10'

SERVING
4

INGREDIENTS

- 3 tbsp. olive oil, divided
- 2 small onions, finely chopped
- 1 jalapeño pepper, minced
- 3/4 cup carrot, grated
- 3/4 cup cabbage, finely chopped
- 11/2 cups quick-cooking oats
- 3/4 cup brown rice, cooked
- 3/4 cup water
- 1/2 cup whole-wheat flour
- 1 large egg
- 1 large egg white
- 1 tsp. baking soda
- 1/4 tsp. cayenne pepper

DIRECTIONS

1. Warm 2 tsp. oil in an average skillet over medium heat.
2. Sauté the onion, jalapeño, carrot, and cabbage for 4 minutes.
3. While the veggies are cooking, combine the oats, rice, water, flour, eggs, baking soda, and cayenne pepper in a medium bowl until well mixed.
4. Add the cooked vegetables to the mixture and stir to combine.
5. Heat the remaining oil in a large skillet over medium heat.
6. Drop the mixture into the skillet, about 1/3 cup per pancake. Cook for 4 minutes, or until bubbles form on the surface of the pancakes and the edges look cooked, then carefully flip them over.
7. Cook the second sides for 3–5 minutes or until the pancakes are hot and firm.
8. Repeat with the remaining mixture and serve.

NUTRIENTS PER SERVING

- Calories: 323
- Protein: 10 g.
- Fat: 11 g.
- Carb: 48 g.
- Sodium: 366 mg.
- Potassium: 381 mg.
- Phosphorus: 263 mg.

136. Egg and Veggie Fajitas

PREPARATION TIME
20'

COOK TIME
10'

SERVING
4

INGREDIENTS

- 3 large eggs
- 3 egg whites
- 2 tsp. chili powder
- 1 tbsp. unsalted butter
- 1 onion, chopped
- 2 garlic cloves, minced
- 1 jalapeño pepper, minced
- 1 red bell pepper, chopped
- 1 cup frozen corn, thawed and drained
- 8 (6-inch) corn tortillas

DIRECTIONS

1. Whisk the eggs, egg whites, and chili powder in a small bowl until well combined. Set aside.
2. In a large skillet, soften the butter over medium heat.
3. Sauté the onion, garlic, jalapeño, bell pepper, and corn, until the vegetables are tender, 3–4 minutes.
4. Add the beaten egg blend to the skillet. Cook, stirring occasionally, till the eggs form large curds and are set, 3–5 minutes.
5. Meanwhile, soften the corn tortillas as directed on the package.
6. Divide the egg mixture evenly among the softened corn tortillas. Roll the tortillas up and serve.

NUTRIENTS PER SERVING

- Calories: 316
- Protein: 14 g.
- Fat: 14 g.
- Carb: 35 g.
- Sodium: 167 mg.
- Potassium: 408 mg.
- Phosphorus: 287 mg.

137. Vegetable Biryani

PREPARATION TIME
20’

COOK TIME
10’

SERVING
4

INGREDIENTS

- 3 cups of frozen cooked brown rice
- 2 tbsp. olive oil
- 1 onion, diced
- 4 garlic cloves, minced
- 1 tbsp. fresh ginger root, skinned and grated
- 1 cup carrot, grated
- 2 cups chopped cauliflower
- 1 cup frozen baby peas, softened and drained
- 2 tsp. curry powder
- 1 cup low-sodium vegetable broth

DIRECTIONS

1. Heat the olive oil over standard heat in a big pot.
2. Add the garlic, onion, and ginger root and sauté, stirring frequently, until tender-crisp, 2 minutes.
3. Add the carrot, cauliflower, peas, and curry powder and cook for 2 minutes longer.
4. Mix in the vegetable broth and steam. Lower the heat, partially cover the skillet, and steam for 6–7 minutes or until the vegetables are tender.
5. Meanwhile, heat the rice as directed on the package.
6. Stir the rice into the vegetable mixture and serve.

NUTRIENTS PER SERVING

- Calories: 378
- Protein: 8 g.
- Fat: 2 g.
- Carb: 53 g.
- Sodium: 113 mg.
- Potassium: 510 mg.
- Phosphorus: 236 mg.

138. Barley Blueberry Avocado Salad

PREPARATION TIME
15'

COOK TIME
15'

SERVING
4

INGREDIENTS

- 1 medium avocado, peeled and chopped
- 2 cups blueberries
- 1 cup quick-cooking barley
- 3 cups low-sodium vegetable broth
- 3 tbsp. extra-virgin olive oil
- 2 tbsp. lemon juice, freshly squeezed
- 1 tsp. yellow mustard
- 1 tsp. honey
- 1/4 cup crumbled feta cheese

DIRECTIONS

1. In a medium pan, add the barley and vegetable broth, and bring to a simmer.
2. Reduce the heat to low, partially cover the pan, and simmer for 10–12 minutes, or until the barley is tender.
3. Meanwhile, whisk together the olive oil, lemon juice, mustard, and honey in a serving bowl until blended.
4. Drain the barley if necessary and add to the bowl; toss to combine.
5. Add the avocado, blueberries, feta, and toss gently. Serve.

Although avocados are high in potassium you can introduce them to your diet limiting the portion to 1/4 of an avocado.

NUTRIENTS PER SERVING

- Calories: 345
- Protein: 7 g.
- Fat: 16 g.
- Carb: 44 g.
- Sodium: 259 mg.
- Potassium: 313 mg.
- Phosphorus: 152 mg.

139. Pasta With Creamy Broccoli Sauce

PREPARATION TIME

20'

COOK TIME

10'

SERVING

4

INGREDIENTS

- 1 lb. broccoli florets
- 1/2 lb. whole-wheat spaghetti pasta
- 3 garlic cloves, halved
- 1 cup low-sodium vegetable broth
- 4 oz. cream cheese
- 1/2 cup grated Parmesan cheese
- 1 tsp. basil leaves, dried
- 2 tbsp. olive oil

DIRECTIONS

1. Boil water in a large saucepan.
2. Meanwhile, warm a big skillet over moderate temperature and add the olive oil. Sauté the broccoli and garlic, stirring frequently, for 3 minutes.
3. Mix the broth to the skillet and steam. Reduce the heat to low, partially cover the skillet, and simmer until the broccoli is tender about 5–6 minutes.
4. Cook the pasta according to package directions. Drain when al dente, reserving 1 cup pasta water.
5. When the broccoli is tender, add the cream cheese and basil. Purée using an immersion blender.
6. You can spoon the assortment into a blender or food processor, about half at a time, and purée until smooth, and transfer the sauce back into the skillet.
7. Add the cooked pasta to the broccoli sauce. Toss, adding enough pasta water until the sauce coats the pasta completely. Sprinkle with the Parmesan and serve.

NUTRIENTS PER SERVING

- Calories: 302
- Protein: 12 g.
- Fat: 14 g.
- Carb: 36 g.
- Sodium: 260 mg.
- Potassium: 375 mg.
- Phosphorus: 223 mg.

140. Asparagus Fried Rice

PREPARATION TIME
20'

COOK TIME
10'

SERVING
4

INGREDIENTS

- 3 large eggs, beaten
- 1/2 tsp. ground ginger
- 2 tsp. low-sodium soy sauce
- 2 tbsp. olive oil
- 1 onion, diced
- 4 garlic cloves, minced
- 1 cup mushrooms, sliced cremini
- 1 (10 oz.) package frozen brown rice, thawed
- 8 oz. fresh asparagus, about 15 spears, cut into 1-inch pieces
- 1 tsp. sesame oil

DIRECTIONS

1. Whisk the eggs, ginger, and soy sauce in a small bowl and set aside.
2. Heat the olive oil in a medium skillet or wok over medium heat.
3. Add the onion and garlic and sauté for 2 minutes until tender-crisp.
4. Add the mushrooms and rice; stir-fry for 3 minutes longer.
5. Put the asparagus and pan-fry for 2 minutes.
6. Move the rice mixture to one side of the skillet and pour in the egg mixture. Stir the eggs until cooked through, 2–3 minutes, and stir into the rice mixture.
7. Sprinkle the fried rice with the sesame oil and serve.

NUTRIENTS PER SERVING

- Calories: 247
- Protein: 9 g.
- Fat: 13 g.
- Carb: 25 g.
- Sodium: 149 mg.
- Potassium: 367 mg.
- Phosphorus: 206 mg.

141. Tex-Mex Pepper Stir-Fry

PREPARATION TIME
20'

COOK TIME
10'

SERVING
4

INGREDIENTS

- 2 cups cooked brown rice
- 1 onion, chopped
- 4 garlic cloves, minced
- 1 jalapeño pepper, minced
- 1 red bell pepper, chopped
- 1 yellow bell pepper, chopped
- 1 cup canned no-salt-added or low-sodium black beans, rinsed and drained
- 1/2 cup Powerhouse Salsa
- Juice from 1 lemon
- 2 tbsp. olive oil

DIRECTIONS

1. Heat the oil in a big skillet over medium-high heat.
2. Add the onion and garlic and stir-fry for 2 minutes.
3. Stir in the jalapeño pepper, red bell pepper, and yellow bell pepper, and stir-fry for another 3 minutes.
4. Add the black beans and stir-fry for 3–5 minutes longer or until the ingredients are heated through.
5. Stir in the salsa and lemon juice and serve over the rice.

NUTRIENTS PER SERVING

- Calories: 297
- Protein: 8 g.
- Fat: 8 g.
- Carb: 49 g.
- Sodium: 29 mg.
- Potassium: 589 mg.
- Phosphorus: 212 mg.

142. Vegetarian Taco Salad

PREPARATION TIME

20'

COOK TIME

0'

SERVING

4

INGREDIENTS

- 1 1/2 cups canned low-sodium or no-salt-added pinto beans, rinsed and drained
- 1 (10 oz.) package frozen brown rice, thawed
- 1 red bell pepper, chopped
- 3 scallions, white and green parts, chopped
- 1 jalapeño pepper, minced
- 1 cup frozen corn, thawed and drained
- 1 tbsp. chili powder
- 1 cup romaine lettuce, chopped
- 2 cups butter lettuce, chopped
- 1/2 cup prepared salsa
- 1/2 cup pepper Jack cheese, grated

DIRECTIONS

1. In a medium bowl, combine the beans, rice, bell pepper, scallions, jalapeño, and corn.
2. Sprinkle with the chili powder and stir gently. Stir in the romaine and butter lettuce.
3. Serve topped with salsa and cheese.

NUTRIENTS PER SERVING

- Calories: 254
- Protein: 11 g.
- Fat: 7 g.
- Carb: 39 g.
- Sodium: 440 mg.
- Potassium: 599 mg.
- Phosphorus: 240 mg.

143. Creamy Red Pepper Pasta

PREPARATION TIME

15'

COOK TIME

15'

SERVING

6

INGREDIENTS

- 12 oz. whole-wheat fettuccine pasta
- 1 leek, white and green parts, cleaned and chopped
- 2 garlic cloves, minced
- 2 large red bell peppers, thinly sliced
- 1 cup low-sodium vegetable broth
- 1 (8 oz.) package cream cheese, softened
- 1 tsp. marjoram leaves, dried
- 2 tbsp. Parmesan cheese, grated
- 2 tbsp. olive oil

DIRECTIONS

1. Boil a large pot of water.
2. Meanwhile, heat the olive oil over average heat in a large skillet.
3. Add the leek, garlic, and bell peppers; sauté for 3–4 minutes or until tender.
4. Stir in the broth and simmer for 2 minutes.
5. Add the pasta to the boiling water and cook until al dente according to package directions. Drain, reserving 1 cup pasta water.
6. Stir the cream cheese and the marjoram into the bell pepper mixture. Purée using an immersion blender.
7. You can also purée this sauce in batches in a blender or food processor. If you choose that method, return all the sauce to the skillet.
8. Add the cooked and drained pasta to the sauce along with enough reserved pasta water to make a smooth sauce that coats the pasta.
9. Sprinkle with the Parmesan cheese and serve.

NUTRIENTS PER SERVING

- Calories: 408
- Protein: 12 g.
- Fat: 19 g.
- Carb: 51 g.
- Sodium: 188 mg.
- Potassium: 330 mg.
- Phosphorus: 222 mg.

144. Herbed Mushroom Burgers

PREPARATION TIME
20'

COOK TIME
10'

SERVING
4

INGREDIENTS

- 4 (4 oz.) cans no-salt-added mushroom pieces and stems, drained
- 4 whole-wheat hamburger buns, split and toasted
- 3 scallions, white and green parts, cut into 1-inch pieces
- 2 garlic cloves, sliced
- 1 tsp. dried Italian seasoning
- 1 large egg
- 2/3 cup rice cereal, crushed puffed
- 2 tbsp. grated Parmesan cheese
- 2 tbsp. olive oil
- 1 tbsp. flour
- 1 cup low-sodium vegetable broth

DIRECTIONS

1. Combine the drained mushrooms, scallions, garlic, and Italian seasoning in a blender or food processor and blend or process until finely sliced.
2. Bring the mushroom mix to a medium bowl. Add the egg, crushed puffed rice cereal, and Parmesan cheese and mix.
3. Form the mixture into four 1/2-inch thick patties and place aside.
4. Heat olive oil in a big skillet above medium temperature.
5. Add the patties and cook, turning once carefully, for 3–4 minutes per side until hot, 160°F internal temperature.
6. Carefully remove the patties from the skillet to a plate and cover with foil to keep warm.
7. Add the flour to the drippings in the skillet and cook, stirring, for 1 minute. Stir in the broth and cook for 2–3 minutes longer or until the sauce thickens and bubbles.
8. On the buns, put the burger and serve with the sauce poured over.

NUTRIENTS PER SERVING

- Calories: 253
- Protein: 11 g.
- Fat: 11 g.
- Carb: 30 g.
- Sodium: 305 mg.
- Potassium: 315 mg.
- Phosphorus: 218 mg.

145. Chickpea Curry

PREPARATION TIME
20'

COOK TIME
10'

SERVING
4

INGREDIENTS

- 1 cup cauliflower florets, chopped
- 2 cups brown rice, cooked
- 2 tbsp. olive oil
- 1 onion, chopped
- 3 garlic cloves, minced
- 1 tbsp. curry powder
- 1 (15 oz.) canned no-salt-added or low-sodium chickpeas, rinsed and drained
- 1 cup low-sodium vegetable broth
- 1 tbsp. lemon juice, freshly squeezed
- Pinch salt
- 1 cup unsweetened almond milk
- 2 tbsp. cornstarch

DIRECTIONS

1. Heat olive oil in a large pot.
2. Mix the garlic and onion and stir-fry for 2–3 minutes or until tender-crisp.
3. Add the cauliflower, curry powder, and chickpeas; sauté for 1 minute.
4. Add the broth, lemon juice, and salt and bring to a simmer. Lower the heat and simmer for 5–6 minutes or until the vegetables are tender.
5. In a small container, mix the milk and cornstarch. Add this mixture to the skillet and cook, stirring constantly, for 2 minutes or until the sauce thickens and comes to a boil.
6. Serve the curry over the rice.

NUTRIENTS PER SERVING

- Calories: 386
- Protein: 12 g.
- Fat: 12 g.
- Carb: 60 g.
- Sodium: 137 mg.
- Potassium: 425 mg.
- Phosphorus: 232 mg.

CHAPTER 22

Snacks and Sides

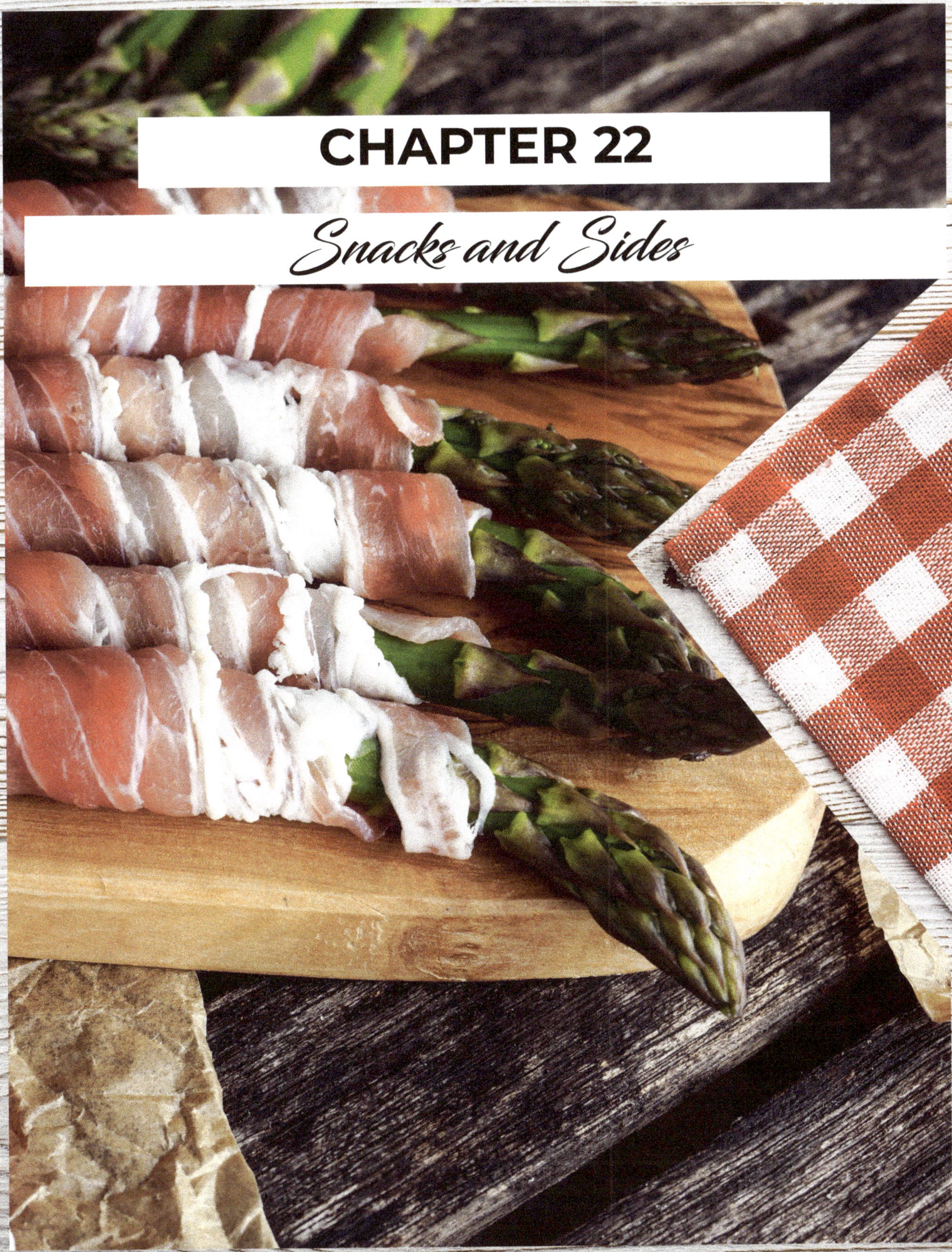

146. Date and Blueberry Muffins

PREPARATION TIME
20'

COOK TIME
30'

SERVING

12 (1 SERVING = 1 MUFFIN)

INGREDIENTS

- 2 tbsp. flax meal
- 6 tbsp. water
- 1 cup almond flour
- 1 cup coconut flour
- 2 tsp. baking soda
- 1 tsp. sea salt
- 2 tbsp. mixed spice
- 1 cup dates, pitted
- 2 cups canned pumpkin
- 1 tsp. lemon juice
- 1/4 cup coconut oil
- 5 oz. frozen blueberries
- 3/4 cup zucchini, grated
- 3/4 cup chopped walnuts

DIRECTIONS

1. Preheat oven to 350°F.
2. Line 12 muffin cups with paper liners.
3. Mix the flax meal and water and leave for a few minutes until it becomes a gel-like consistency.
4. Mix almond flour, coconut flour, baking soda, sea salt, and mixed spice in a large bowl. Set aside.
5. In a food processor, pulse together the pitted dates, pumpkin, and lemon juice together with the flax water and coconut oil.
6. Add the pumpkin mix into the dry ingredients. Mix well.
7. Gently stir in the blueberries, grated zucchini, and walnuts.
8. Divide the mixture evenly between the prepared muffin cups.
9. Bake for about 30 minutes. If the muffins are too gooey, after this time, leave for a few minutes longer.

NUTRIENTS PER SERVING

- Calories: 211
- Protein: 5 g.
- Fat: 12 g.
- Carb 23.3 g.
- Sodium: 129 mg.
- Potassium: 227 mg.
- Phosphorus: 316 mg.

147. Cranberry Orange Cookies

PREPARATION TIME
10'

COOK TIME
1 HOUR

SERVING
36

INGREDIENTS

- 4 cups all-purpose white flour
- 2 1/2 tsp. baking powder
- 2 sticks unsalted butter
- 4 eggs
- 3 tsp. grated orange zest
- 1 1/2 cup sugar
- 1/2 tsp. salt
- 1/2 macadamia nuts, chopped
- 1/2 cup cranberries, dried

DIRECTIONS

1. Preheat oven to 350°F.
2. Prepare the cookie sheets with parchment paper.
3. In a bowl sift together flour, salt, and baking powder.
4. In a large bowl beat sugar, butter, orange zest, and salt with a mixer. Add eggs, until well mixed and melted. Slowly add flour mixture and mix until well combined.
5. Add macadamia nuts and cranberries into dough.
6. Remove dough from the bowl onto a very lightly floured surface, form dough into a loaf.
7. Place on a baking sheet and bake for about 40 minutes until lightly golden on the surface. Remove from oven cool loaf for half an hour.
8. Cut the loaf into slices using a knife. Place slices back on the baking sheet and bake for another 15–20 minutes until a nice golden brown. Take away from the oven and cool on a cooling rack.
9. Serve and enjoy!

NUTRIENTS PER SERVING (=1 COOKIE)

- Calories: 152
- Protein: 2 g.
- Fat: 7 g.
- Carb: 21 g.
- Sodium: 75 mg.
- Potassium: 29 mg.
- Phosphorus: 35 mg.

148. No-Bake Oat Cookies

PREPARATION TIME
30'

COOK TIME
0

SERVING
24

INGREDIENTS

- 1/2 cup plain soymilk
- 1 3/4 cups sugar
- 1/2 cup vegan butter
- 1 tsp. vanilla extract
- 3 1/2 cups quick-cooking oats
- 1/4 cup unsweetened cocoa powder
- 1/2 cup peanut butter, smooth or crunchy

DIRECTIONS

1. In a small pot mix the milk, butter, sugar, peanut butter, and vanilla and cook until smooth and creamy.
2. In a large bowl combine the oats and cocoa powder.
3. Pour the warm milk mixture over the oats and stir until all the ingredients have been combined.
4. Place dollops of mixture onto a waxed paper-lined cookie sheet and let cool for about half an hour.

NUTRIENTS PER SERVING

- Calories: 171
- Protein: 3.3 g.
- Fat: 6.7 g.
- Carb: 25.5 g.
- Sodium: 119 mg.
- Potassium: 287 mg.
- Phosphorus: 216 mg.

149. Chocolate Coconut Quinoa Slices

PREPARATION TIME
10'

COOK TIME
25

SERVING
12

INGREDIENTS

- 3/4 cup quinoa
- 1/2 cup dates, dried chopped
- 3 tbsp. maple syrup
- 2 tbsp. olive oil
- 2 tbsp. ground flaxseed
- 1/2 tsp. almond extract
- 1/4 tsp. salt
- 1/2 cup chocolate protein powder
- 1/2 cup whole wheat flour
- 1/4 cup vegan chocolate chips
- 1/4 cup shredded coconut water

DIRECTIONS

1. Preheat the oven to 350°F.
2. Prepare an 8x8 ovenproof baking dish. Grease lightly with oil.
3. Rinse the quinoa in cold water and leave to soak for about 10 minutes.
4. Drain the quinoa. Place 1 cup of water in a small saucepan bring to boil. Add the quinoa and simmer over low heat for about 12 minutes. Cool.
5. Mix the cooked quinoa, dates, maple syrup, olive oil, flaxseed, almond extract, and salt in a food processor.
6. Process until fairly smooth.
7. In a separate bowl stir together the chocolate protein powder, flour, chocolate chips, and coconut.
8. Fold the dry mixture into the wet mixture with a flat spatula or knife.
9. Press into the prepared baking dish. Even out the top.
10. Bake for about 25 minutes, until firm.
11. Cool and then slice into bars.
12. Stock in a sealed basin for about 1 week or freeze up to 3 months.

NUTRIENTS PER SERVING

- Calories: 160
- Protein: 9 g.
- Fat: 4.7 g.
- Carb: 22.4 g.
- Sodium: 123 mg.
- Potassium: 227 mg.
- Phosphorus: 219 mg.

150. Pineapple Raspberry Parfaits

PREPARATION TIME
6'

COOK TIME
0

SERVING
2

INGREDIENTS

- 1/2 pint fresh raspberries
- 1 1/2 cup fresh or frozen pineapple chunks
- 2 containers (8 oz. each) non-fat peach yogurt

DIRECTIONS

1. In a parfait glass, layer the yogurt, raspberries, and pineapples alternately. Chill inside the refrigerator.
2. Serve chilled.

NUTRIENTS PER SERVING

- Calories: 319
- Protein: 22 g.
- Fat: 1 g.
- Carb: 60 g.
- Sodium: 85 mg.
- Potassium: 479 mg.
- Phosphorus: 93 mg.

151. Cinnamon Apple Chips

PREPARATION TIME
5'

COOK TIME
3 HOURS

SERVING
4

INGREDIENTS

- 4 apples
- 1 tsp. ground cinnamon

DIRECTIONS

1. Preheat the oven to 200°F. Line a baking sheet with parchment paper.
2. Slice the apples into 1/8-inch slices. Toss your cinnamon and apple slices to coat.
3. In a single layer, spread the apples on the prepared baking sheet.
4. Cook for 2–3 hours, until the apples are dry. They will still be soft while hot but will crisp once completely cooled.
5. Save in a sealed container for 4 days.

NUTRIENTS PER SERVING

- Calories: 96
- Protein: 1 g.
- Fat: 0 g.
- Carb: 26 g.
- Sodium: 2 mg.
- Potassium: 198 mg.
- Phosphorus: 0 mg.

152. Spiced Pumpkin Pancakes

PREPARATION TIME
5'

COOK TIME
6'

SERVING
2

INGREDIENTS

- 1 cup of canned pumpkin, no added salt or sugar
- 2 tbsp. water
- 3 egg whites
- 1 tsp. paprika
- 1 tsp. cayenne pepper
- 1 tsp. cinnamon
- 1 tbsp. coconut oil

DIRECTIONS

1. Blend the pumpkin flesh with water to form a smooth pulp.
2. Now add the rest of the ingredients (minus the coconut oil) and mix well.
3. Heat coconut oil in a large skillet.
4. Pour the pumpkin mixture into the pan into individual rounded pancakes (go easy at first and pour your mixture into little circles, keep pouring whilst tilting the pan until you have a pancake to your desired shape).
5. Lift the mixture with a spatula and then flip. Cook for 3 minutes on either side.
6. Serve warm; they taste great with sweet or savory accompaniments.

NUTRIENTS PER SERVING

- Calories: 125
- Protein: 5 g.
- Fat: 8 g.
- Carb: 13 g.
- Sodium: 298 mg.
- Potassium: 355 mg.
- Phosphorus: 55 mg.

153. Roasted Mint Carrots

PREPARATION TIME
5'

COOK TIME
20'

SERVING
6

INGREDIENTS

- 1 lb. carrots, trimmed
- 1 tbsp. extra-virgin olive oil
- Freshly ground black pepper
- 1/4 cup mint, thinly sliced

DIRECTIONS

1. Preheat the oven to 425°F.
2. In a single layer, arrange the carrots on a rimmed baking sheet. Sprinkle with the olive oil and shake the carrots on the sheet to coat.
3. Season with pepper. Roast for 20 minutes, or until tender and browned, stirring twice while cooking. Sprinkle with the mint and serve.

NUTRIENTS PER SERVING

- Calories: 51
- Protein: 1 g.
- Fat: 2 g.
- Carb: 7 g.
- Sodium: 52 mg.
- Potassium: 242 mg.
- Phosphorus: 26 mg.

154. Walnut Butter on Cracker

PREPARATION TIME
2'

COOK TIME
0'

SERVING
1

INGREDIENTS

- 1 tbsp. walnut butter
- 2 pieces Mary's gone crackers

DIRECTIONS

1. Spread 1/2 tbsp. of walnut butter per cracker and enjoy.

NUTRIENTS PER SERVING

- Calories: 134
- Protein: 1 g.
- Fat: 14 g.
- Carb: 4 g.
- Sodium: 138 mg.
- Potassium: 11 mg.
- Phosphorus: 19 mg.

155. Savory Collard Chips

PREPARATION TIME
5'

COOK TIME
20'

SERVING
4

INGREDIENTS

- 1 bunch collard greens
- 1 tsp. extra-virgin olive oil
- Juice of 1/2 lemon
- 1/2 tsp. garlic powder
- 1/4 tsp. freshly ground black pepper

DIRECTIONS

1. Preheat the oven to 350°F. Line a baking sheet with parchment paper.
2. Cut the collards into 2-by-2-inch squares and pat dry with paper towels. In a large container, mix the greens with the olive oil, lemon juice, garlic powder, and pepper.
3. Use your hands to mix well, massaging the dressing into the greens until evenly coated.
4. Arrange the collards in a single layer on the baking sheet and cook for 8 minutes. Turn over the pieces and cook for an additional 8 minutes, until crisp.
5. Remove from the oven, let cool, and store in an airtight container in a cool location for up to three days.

NUTRIENTS PER SERVING

- Calories: 24
- Protein: 1 g.
- Fat: 1 g.
- Carb: 3 g.
- Sodium: 8 mg.
- Potassium: 72 mg.
- Phosphorus: 6 mg.

156. Choco-Chip Cookies

PREPARATION TIME
15’

COOK TIME
15’

SERVING
24

INGREDIENTS

- 1 cup almond flour
- 1/2 cup unsalted butter
- 1 large egg
- 1/2 cup brown sugar
- 1/2 tsp. vanilla extract
- 1/2 tsp. baking soda
- 1/2 salt
- 1 cup semisweet Choco chip

DIRECTIONS

1. Preheat oven to 375°F and grease baking sheets with cooking spray.
2. In a medium bowl, whisk the flour, baking soda, and salt.
3. In a large bowl, with a mixer beat butter until well combined. Add brown sugar and mixing continuously until creamy.
4. Mix in vanilla and egg and beat for a minute. Cup by cup mix in the dry ingredients until well incorporated.
5. Fold in choco-chips. Get a tbsp. full of the batter and roll with your moistened hands into a morsel.
6. Evenly place morsels into prepped baking sheets. Place in the oven and bake for 15 minutes or until golden brown.
7. Remove from oven, cool on a wire rack.
8. Cookies can be stored for up to 2-weeks in a tightly sealed container or longer in the ref.

NUTRIENTS PER SERVING

- Calories: 110
- Protein: 2 g.
- Fat: 7 g.
- Carb: 13 g.
- Sodium: 85 mg.
- Potassium: 65 mg.
- Phosphorus: 30 mg.

157. Lemon and Parsley Coleslaw

PREPARATION TIME
15'

COOK TIME
0'

SERVING
2

INGREDIENTS

- 1 carrot, peeled and finely sliced
- 1 cup white cabbage, peeled and finely sliced
- 1 lemon, juice, and zest
- 1 tbsp. fresh parsley, finely chopped
- 1 tbsp. extra virgin olive oil

DIRECTIONS

1. Soak vegetables in warm water for 5–10 minutes.
2. Drain and rinse with cold water.
3. Combine with the rest of the ingredients, cover, and cool in the refrigerator before serving.

NUTRIENTS PER SERVING

- Calories: 89
- Protein: 1 g.
- Fat: 7 g.
- Carb: 7 g.
- Sodium: 30 mg.
- Potassium: 208 mg.
- Phosphorus: 25 mg.

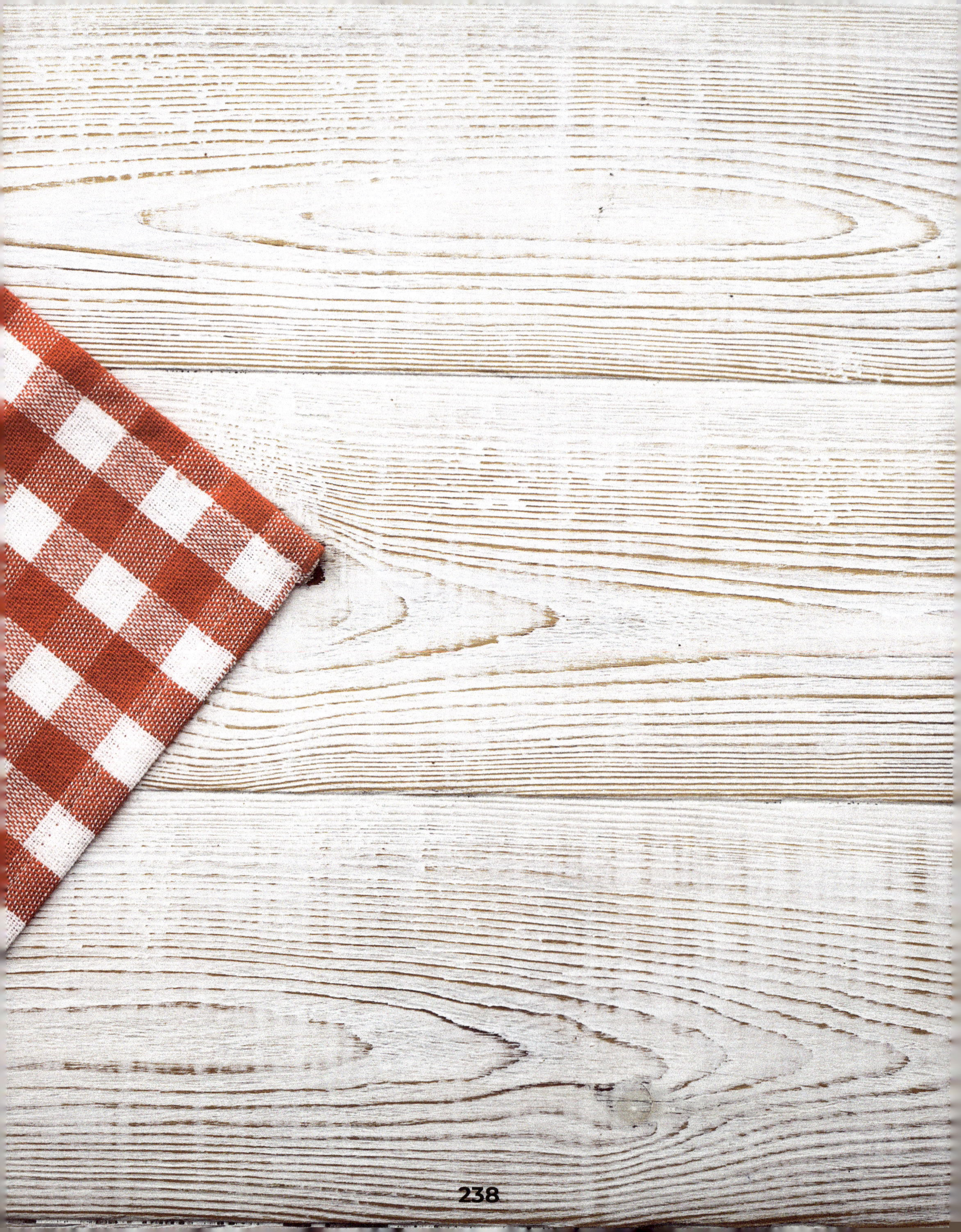

CHAPTER 23

Dessert Recipes

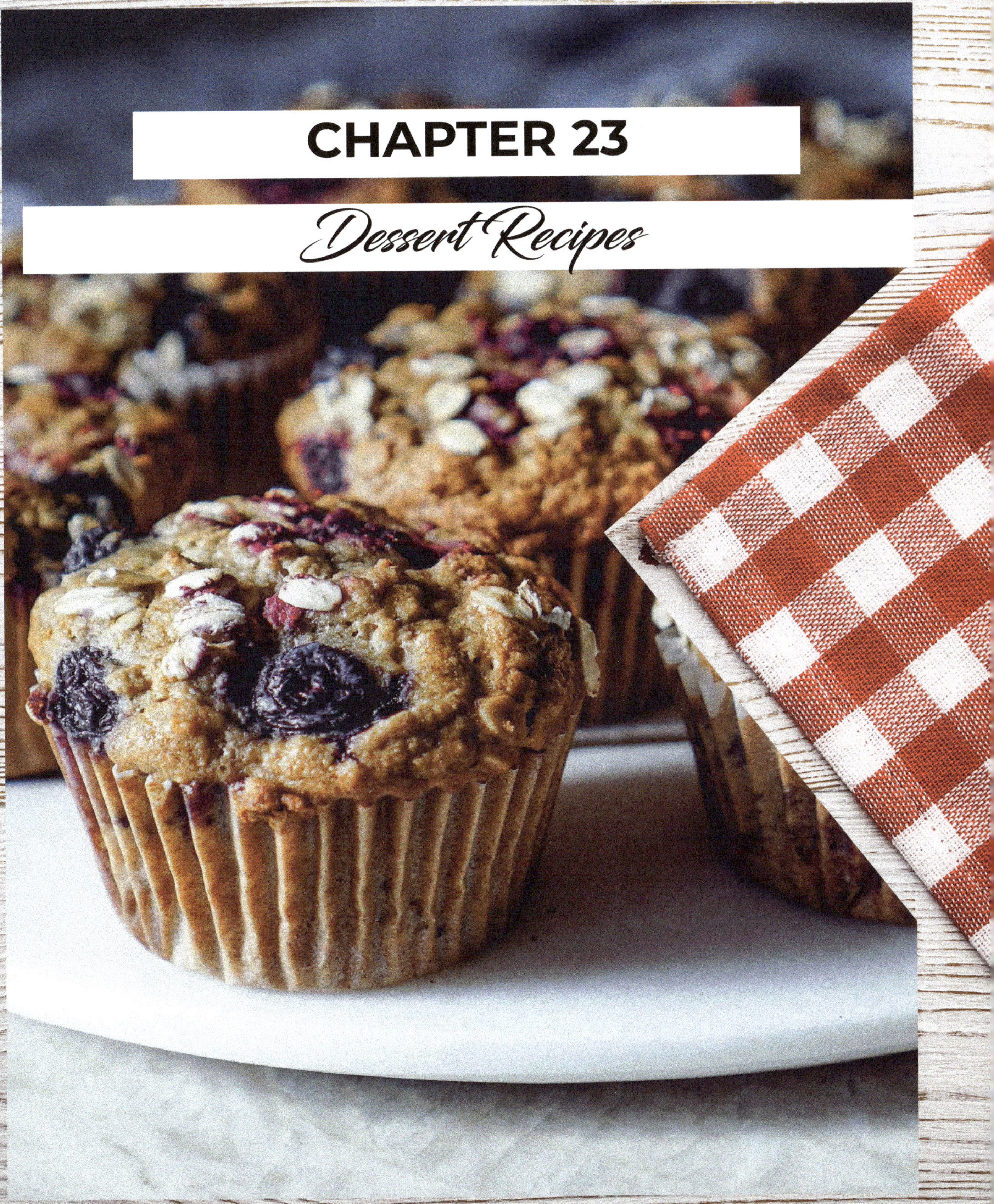

158. Chocolate Trifle

PREPARATION TIME
20’

COOK TIME
15’

SERVING
4

INGREDIENTS

- 1 small plain sponge Swiss roll
- 3 oz. custard powder
- 5 oz. hot water
- 16 oz. canned mandarins
- 3 tbsp. sherry
- 5 oz. double cream
- 4 chocolate squares, grated

DIRECTIONS

1. Whisk the custard powder with water in a bowl until dissolved.
2. In a bowl, mix the custard well until it becomes creamy and let it sit for 15 minutes.
3. Spread the Swiss roll and cut it into 4 squares.
4. Place the Swiss roll in the 4 serving cups.
5. Top the Swiss roll with mandarin, custard, cream, and chocolate.
6. Serve.

NUTRIENTS PER SERVING

- Calories: 315
- Protein: 2.9 g.
- Fat: 13.5 g.
- Sodium: 185 mg.
- Potassium: 129 mg.
- Phosphorus: 184 mg.

159. Pineapple Meringues

PREPARATION TIME

10'

COOK TIME

0'

SERVING

4

INGREDIENTS

- 4 meringue nests
- 8 oz. crème Fraiche
- 2 oz. stem ginger, chopped
- 8 oz. can pineapple chunks

DIRECTIONS

1. Place the meringue nests on the serving plates.
2. Whisk the ginger with crème Fraiche and pineapple chunks.
3. Divide the pineapple mixture over the meringue nests.
4. Serve.

NUTRIENTS PER SERVING

- Calories: 312
- Protein: 2.3 g.
- Sodium: 41 mg.
- Potassium: 110 mg.
- Phosphorus: 104 mg.

160. Baked Custard

PREPARATION TIME
15'

COOK TIME
30'

SERVING
1

INGREDIENTS

- 1/2 cup milk
- 1 egg, beaten
- 1/8 tsp. nutmeg
- 1/8 tsp. vanilla
- Sweetener, to taste
- 1/2 cup water

DIRECTIONS

1. Lightly warm up the milk in a pan, then whisk in the egg, nutmeg, vanilla, and sweetener.
2. Pour this custard mixture into a ramekin.
3. Place the ramekin in a baking pan and pour 1/2 cup water into the pan.
4. Bake the custard for 30 minutes at 325°F.
5. Serve fresh.

NUTRIENTS PER SERVING

- Calories: 127
- Fat: 7 g.
- Sodium: 119 mg.
- Potassium: 171 mg.
- Phosphorus: 309 mg.

161. Strawberry Pie

PREPARATION TIME
15'

COOK TIME
25'

SERVING
6

INGREDIENTS

- 1 unbaked pie shell (9 inches)
- 4 cups strawberries, fresh
- 1 cup brown Swerve
- 3 tbsp. arrowroot powder
- 2 tbsp. lemon juice
- 8 tbsp. whipped cream topping

DIRECTIONS

1. Spread the pie shell in the pie pan and bake it until golden brown.
2. Now mash 2 cups of strawberries with lemon juice, arrowroot powder, and Swerve in a bowl.
3. Add the mixture to a saucepan and cook on moderate heat until it thickens.
4. Allow the mixture to cool then spread it in the pie shell.
5. Slice the remaining strawberries and spread them over the pie filling.
6. Refrigerate for 1 hour then garnish with whipped cream.
7. Serve fresh and enjoy.

NUTRIENTS PER SERVING

- Calories: 236
- Protein: 2.2 g.
- Fat: 11.1 g.
- Sodium: 183 mg.
- Potassium: 178 mg.
- Phosphorus: 47.2 mg.

162. Apple Crisp

PREPARATION TIME

20'

COOK TIME

45'

SERVING

6

INGREDIENTS

- 4 cups apples, peeled and chopped
- 1/2 tsp. stevia
- 3 tbsp. brandy
- 2 tsp. lemon juice
- 1/2 tsp. cinnamon
- 1/8 tsp. nutmeg
- 3/4 cup dry oats
- 1/4 cup brown Swerve
- 2 tbsp. flour
- 2 tbsp. butter

DIRECTIONS

1. Toss the oats with the flour, butter, and brown Swerve in a bowl and keep it aside.
2. Whisk the remaining crisp ingredients in an 8-inch baking pan.
3. Spread the oats mixture over the crispy filling.
4. Bake it for 45 minutes at 350°F in a preheated oven.
5. Slice and serve.

NUTRIENTS PER SERVING

- Calories: 214
- Protein: 2.1 g.
- Fat: 4.8 g.
- Sodium: 48 mg.
- Potassium: 212 mg.
- Phosphorus: 348 mg.

163. Almond Cookies

PREPARATION TIME
10'

COOK TIME
12'

SERVING
24

INGREDIENTS

- 1 cup butter, softened
- 1 cup granulate Swerve
- 1 egg
- 3 cups flour
- 1 tsp. baking soda
- 1 tsp. almond extract

DIRECTIONS

1. Beat the butter with the Swerve in a mixer then gradually stir in the remaining ingredients.
2. Mix well until it forms a cookie dough then divide the dough into small balls.
3. Spread each ball into 3/4 inch rounds and place them on a cookie sheet.
4. Poke 2–3 holes in each cookie then bake for 12 minutes at 400°F.
5. Serve.

NUTRIENTS PER SERVING

- Calories: 159
- Protein: 1.9 g.
- Fat: 7.9 g
- Sodium: 144 mg.
- Potassium: 23 mg.
- Phosphorus: 274 mg.

164. Lime Pie

PREPARATION TIME
10'

COOK TIME
5'

SERVING
8

INGREDIENTS

- 5 tbsp. butter, unsalted
- 1 1/4 cups breadcrumbs
- 1/4 cup granulated Swerve
- 1/3 cup lime juice
- 14 oz. condensed milk
- 1 cup heavy whipping cream
- 1 pie shell (9 inches)

DIRECTIONS

1. Switch on your gas oven and preheat it to 350ªF.
2. Whisk the cracker crumbs with the Swerve and melted butter in a suitable bowl.
3. Spread this cracker crumbs crust in a 9 inches' pie shell and bake it for 5 minutes.
4. Meanwhile, mix the condensed milk with the lime juice in a bowl.
5. Whisk the heavy cream in a mixer until foamy, then add in the condensed milk mixture.
6. Mix well, then spread this filling in the baked crust.
7. Refrigerate the pie for 4 hours.
8. Slice and serve.

NUTRIENTS PER SERVING

- Calories: 391
- Protein: 5.3 g.
- Fat: 22.4 g.
- Sodium: 52 mg.
- Potassium: 221 mg.
- Phosphorus: 199 mg.

165. Buttery Lemon Squares

PREPARATION TIME
10'

COOK TIME
35'

SERVING
12

INGREDIENTS

- 1 cup refined Swerve
- 1 cup flour
- 1/2 cup butter, unsalted
- 1 cup granulated Swerve
- 1/2 tsp. baking powder
- 2 eggs, beaten
- 4 tbsp. lemon juice
- 1 tbsp. butter, unsalted, softened
- 1 tbsp. lemon zest

DIRECTIONS

1. Start mixing 1/4 cup refined Swerve, 1/2 cup butter, and flour in a bowl.
2. Spread this crust mixture in an 8-inch square pan and press it.
3. Bake this flour crust for 15 minutes at 350°F.
4. Meanwhile, prepare the filling by beating 2 tbsp. lemon juice, granulated Swerve, eggs, lemon rind, and baking powder in a mixer.
5. Spread this filling in the baked crust and bake again for about 20 minutes.
6. Meanwhile, prepare the squares icing by beating 2 tbsp. lemon juice, 1 tbsp. butter, and 3/4 cup refined Swerve.
7. Once the lemon pie is baked well, allow it to cool.
8. Sprinkle the icing mixture on top of the lemon pie then cut it into 36 squares.
9. Serve.

NUTRIENTS PER SERVING

- Calories: 229
- Protein: 2.1 g.
- Fat: 9.5 g.
- Sodium: 66 mg.
- Potassium: 51 mg.
- Phosphorus: 257 mg.

166. Blackberry Cream Cheese Pie

PREPARATION TIME
15'

COOK TIME
45'

SERVING
8

INGREDIENTS

- 1/3 cup butter, unsalted
- 4 cups blackberries
- 1 tsp. stevia
- 1 cup flour
- 1/2 tsp. baking powder
- 3/4 cup cream cheese

DIRECTIONS

1. Switch your gas oven to 375°F to preheat.
2. Layer a 2 1/4 baking dish with melted butter.
3. Mix the blackberries with stevia in a small bowl.
4. Beat the remaining ingredients in a mixer until they form a smooth batter.
5. Evenly spread this pie batter in the prepared baking dish and top it with blackberries.
6. Bake the blackberry pie for about 45 minutes in the preheated oven.
7. Slice and serve once chilled.

NUTRIENTS PER SERVING

- Calories: 239
- Protein: 2.8 g.
- Fat: 8.4 g.
- Sodium: 63 mg.
- Potassium: 170 mg.
- Phosphorus: 105 mg.

167. Apple Cinnamon Pie

PREPARATION TIME
20'

COOK TIME
50'

SERVING
12

INGREDIENTS

Apple filling:

- 9 cups apples, peeled, cored, and sliced
- 1 tbsp. stevia
- 1/3 cup all-purpose flour
- 2 tbsp. lemon juice
- 1 tsp. ground cinnamon
- 2 tbsp. butter

Pie dough:

- 2 1/4 cups all-purpose flour
- 1 tsp. stevia
- 1 1/2 sticks unsalted butter
- 6 oz. cream cheese
- 3 tbsp. cold heavy whipping cream
- Water, if needed

DIRECTIONS

1. Start by preheating your gas oven at 425°F.
2. Mix the apple slices with cinnamon, 1 tbsp. of butter, lemon juice, flour, and stevia in a bowl and keep it aside covered.
3. Whisk the flour with stevia, butter, cream cheese, and cream in a mixing bowl to form the dough.
4. If the dough is too dry, slowly add some water to make a smooth dough ball.
5. Cut the dough into two equal-size pieces and spread them into a 9-inch sheet.
6. Place one of the sheets at the bottom of a 9-inch pie pan.
7. Evenly spread the apples in this pie shell and add 1 tbsp. of butter over it.
8. Cover the apple filling with the second sheet of the dough and pinch down the edges.
9. Make 1-inch deep cuts on top of the pie and bake for about 50 minutes until golden.
10. Slice and serve.

NUTRIENTS PER SERVING

- Calories: 303
- Protein: 4.2 g.
- Fat: 8.8 g.
- Sodium: 30 mg.
- Potassium: 229 mg.
- Phosphorus: 381 mg.

168. Maple Crisp Bars

PREPARATION TIME
10'

COOK TIME
15'

SERVING
20

INGREDIENTS

- 1/3 cup butter
- 1 cup brown Swerve
- 1 tsp. maple extract
- 1/2 cup maple syrup
- 8 cups of rice cereal, puffed

DIRECTIONS

1. Mix the butter with Swerve, maple extract, and syrup in a saucepan over moderate heat.
2. Cook by slowly stirring this mixture for 5 minutes then toss in the rice cereal.
3. Mix well, then press this cereal mixture in a 13x9 inches baking dish.
4. Refrigerate the mixture for 2 hours then cut into 20 bars.
5. Serve.

NUTRIENTS PER SERVING

- Calories: 107
- Protein: 0.4 g.
- Fat: 3.1 g.
- Sodium: 36 mg.
- Potassium: 24 mg.
- Phosphorus: 233 mg.

169. Pineapple Gelatin Pie

PREPARATION TIME
10'

COOK TIME
5'

SERVING
8

INGREDIENTS

- 2/3 cup graham cracker crumbs
- 2 1/2 tbsp. butter, melted
- 1 (20 oz.) can crushed pineapple, juice packed
- 1 small gelatin pack
- 1 tbsp. lemon juice
- 2 egg whites, pasteurized
- 1/4 tsp. cream of tartar

DIRECTIONS

1. Whisk the crumbs with the butter in a bowl then spread them onto an 8-inch pie plate.
2. Bake the crust for 5 minutes at 425°F.
3. Meanwhile, mix the pineapple juice with the gelatin in a saucepan.
4. Place it over low heat then add the pineapple and lemon juice. Mix well.
5. Whip the cream of tartar and egg whites in a mixer until creamy.
6. Add the cooked pineapple mixture then mix well.
7. Spread this filling in the baked crust.
8. Refrigerate the pie for 4 hours then slice.
9. Serve.

NUTRIENTS PER SERVING

- Calories: 106
- Protein: 2.2 g.
- Fat: 4.2 g.
- Sodium: 117 mg.
- Potassium: 33 mg.
- Phosphorus: 231 mg.

170. Chocolate Gelatin Mousse

PREPARATION TIME
10'

COOK TIME
5'

SERVING
4

INGREDIENTS

- 1 tsp. stevia
- 1/2 tsp. gelatin
- 1/4 cup milk
- 1/2 cup chocolate chips
- 1 tsp. vanilla
- 1/2 cup heavy cream, whipped

DIRECTIONS

1. Whisk the stevia with the gelatin and milk in a saucepan and cook up to a boil.
2. Stir in the chocolate and vanilla then mix well until it has completely melted.
3. Beat the cream in a mixer until fluffy then fold in the chocolate mixture.
4. Mix it gently with a spatula then transfer to the serving bowl.
5. Refrigerate the dessert for 4 hours.
6. Serve.

NUTRIENTS PER SERVING

- Calories: 200
- Protein: 3.2 g.
- Sodium: 31 mg.
- Potassium: 100 mg.
- Phosphorus: 120 mg.

CHAPTER 24

Smoothies & Drinks

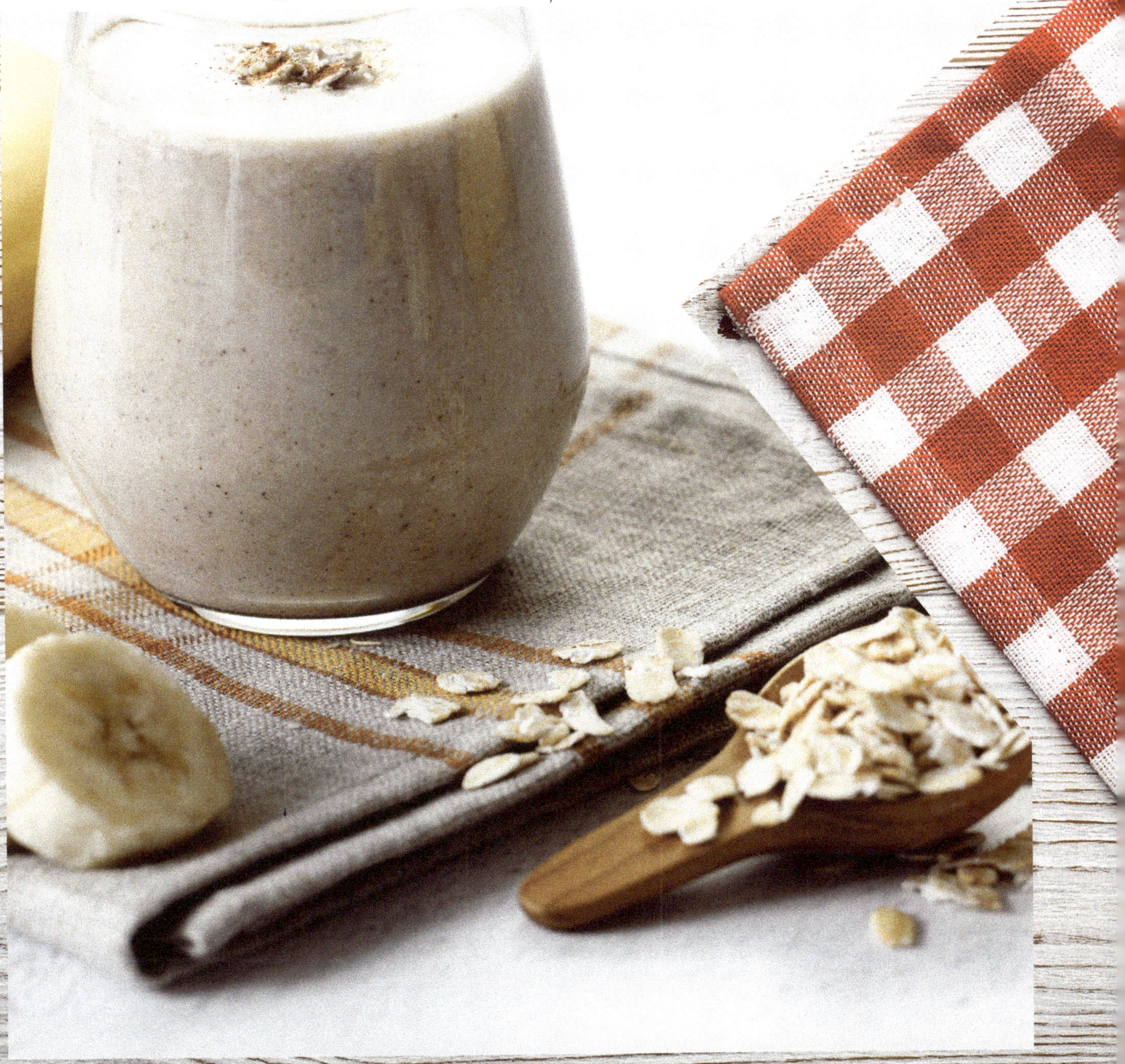

171. Almonds Et Blueberries Smoothie

PREPARATION TIME
5'

COOK TIME
0'

SERVING
2

INGREDIENTS

- 1/4 cup ground almonds, unsalted
- 1 cup fresh blueberries
- 1 lemon fresh juice
- 1 cup fresh kale leaf
- 1/2 cup coconut water
- 1 cup of water
- 2 tbsp. plain yogurt (optional)

DIRECTIONS

1. Dump all ingredients in your high-speed blender, and blend until your smoothie is smooth.
2. Pour the mixture into a chilled glass.
3. Serve and enjoy!

NUTRIENTS PER SERVING

- Calories: 110
- Protein: 2 g.
- Fat: 7 g.
- Carb: 8 g.
- Sodium: 101 mg.
- Potassium: 27 mg.
- Phosphorus: 16 mg.

172. Almonds and Zucchini Smoothie

PREPARATION TIME
5'

COOK TIME
0'

SERVING
2

INGREDIENTS

- 1 cup zucchini, unsalted, cooked, and mashed
- 1 1/2 cups almond milk
- 1 tbsp. almond butter, plain, unsalted
- 1 tsp. pure almond extract
- 2 tbsp. ground almonds or macadamia almonds
- 1/2 cup water
- 1 cup ice cubes crushed (optional, for serving)

DIRECTIONS

1. Dump all ingredients from the list above in your fast-speed blender; blend for 45–60 seconds or to taste.
2. Serve with crushed ice.

NUTRIENTS PER SERVING

- Calories: 322
- Protein: 6 g.
- Fat: 30 g.
- Carb: 6 g.
- Sodium: 121 mg.
- Potassium: 27 mg.
- Phosphorus: 26 mg.

173. Avocado With Walnut Butter Smoothie

PREPARATION TIME

5'

COOK TIME

0'

SERVING

2

INGREDIENTS

- 1 avocado, diced
- 1 cup baby spinach
- 1 cup coconut milk, canned
- 1 tbsp. walnut butter, unsalted
- 2 tbsp. natural sweeteners such as stevia, erythritol, Truvia, etc.

DIRECTIONS

1. Place all ingredients into a food processor or a blender; blend until smooth or to taste.
2. Add more or less walnut butter.
3. Drink and enjoy!

NUTRIENTS PER SERVING

- Calories: 364
- Protein: 8 g.
- Fat: 35 g.
- Carb: 7 g.
- Sodium: 119 mg.
- Potassium: 27 mg.
- Phosphorus: 46 mg.

174. Baby Spinach and Dill Smoothie

PREPARATION TIME
5'

COOK TIME
0'

SERVING
2

INGREDIENTS

- 1 cup of fresh baby spinach leaves
- 2 tbsp. of fresh dill, chopped
- 1 1/2 cup of water
- 1/2 avocado, chopped into cubes
- 1 tbsp. chia seeds (optional)
- 2 tbsp. of natural sweetener stevia or erythritol (optional)

DIRECTIONS

1. Place all ingredients into a fast-speed blender. Beat until smooth and all ingredients united well.
2. Serve and enjoy!

NUTRIENTS PER SERVING

- Calories: 136
- Protein: 7 g.
- Fat: 10 g.
- Carb: 8 g.
- Sodium: 111 mg.
- Potassium: 47 mg.
- Phosphorus: 36 mg.

175. Blueberries and Coconut Smoothie

PREPARATION TIME
5'

COOK TIME
0'

SERVING
5

INGREDIENTS

- 1 cup of frozen blueberries, unsweetened
- 1 cup stevia or erythritol sweetener
- 2 cups coconut milk, canned
- 1 cup of fresh spinach leaves
- 2 tbsp. shredded coconut, unsweetened
- 3/4 cup water

DIRECTIONS

1. Place all ingredients from the list in a food processor or your strong blender.
2. Blend for 45–60 seconds or to taste.
3. Ready to drink! Serve!

NUTRIENTS PER SERVING

- Calories: 190
- Protein: 3 g.
- Fat: 18 g.
- Carb: 8 g.
- Sodium: 129 mg.
- Potassium: 207 mg.
- Phosphorus: 216 mg.

176. Collard Greens and Cucumber Smoothie

PREPARATION TIME
15'

COOK TIME
5'

SERVING
2

INGREDIENTS

- 1 cup collard greens
- A few fresh peppermint leaves
- 1 big cucumber
- 1 lime, freshly juiced
- 1/2 cups avocado sliced
- 1 1/2 cup water
- 1 cup crushed ice
- 1/4 cup of natural sweetener erythritol or stevia (optional)

DIRECTIONS

1. Rinse and clean your collard greens from any dirt.
2. Blend all ingredients in a blender until your smoothie is combined well.
3. Pour in a glass and drink. Enjoy!

NUTRIENTS PER SERVING

- Calories: 123
- Protein: 4 g.
- Fat: 11 g.
- Carb: 8 g.
- Sodium: 123 mg.
- Potassium: 57 mg.
- Phosphorus: 26 mg.

177. Creamy Dandelion Greens and Celery Smoothie

PREPARATION TIME
10'

COOK TIME
0'

SERVING
2

INGREDIENTS

- 1 handful of raw dandelion greens
- 2 celery sticks
- 2 tbsp. chia seeds
- 1 small piece of ginger, minced
- 1/2 cup almond milk
- 1/2 cup of water
- 1/2 cup plain yogurt

DIRECTIONS

1. Rinse and clean dandelion leaves from any dirt; add in a high-speed blender.
2. Clean the ginger; keep only the inner part and cut into small slices; add in a blender.
3. Blend all remaining ingredients until smooth.
4. Serve and enjoy!

NUTRIENTS PER SERVING

- Calories: 58
- Protein: 3 g.
- Fat: 6 g.
- Carb: 5 g.
- Sodium: 125 mg.
- Potassium: 27 mg.
- Phosphorus: 76 mg.

178. Scrumptious Strawberry Smoothie

PREPARATION TIME
5'

COOK TIME
0'

SERVING
2

INGREDIENTS

- 1 cup fresh strawberries, sliced
- 1 cup rice milk, unenriched

DIRECTIONS

1. Blend in a food processor or smoothie maker and serve over ice if desired.
2. Enjoy!

NUTRIENTS PER SERVING

- Calories: 80
- Protein: 4 g.
- Fat: 2 g.
- Carb: 12 g.
- Sodium: 58 mg.
- Potassium: 276 mg.
- Phosphorus: 73 mg.

179. Ginger & Lemon Green Iced-Tea

PREPARATION TIME
5'

COOK TIME
0'

SERVING
2

INGREDIENTS

- 2 cups concentrated green or matcha tea served hot
- 1 lemon, cut into wedges
- 1/4 cup crystallized ginger, chopped into fine pieces

DIRECTIONS

1. Get a glass container and mix the tea with the ginger and then cover and chill for 3 hours.
2. Strain and pour into serving glasses on top of ice if you wish.
3. Garnish with a wedge of lemon to serve.

NUTRIENTS PER SERVING

- Calories: 20
- Protein: 1 g.
- Fat: 0 g.
- Carb: 5 g.
- Sodium: 4 mg.
- Potassium: 106 mg.
- Phosphorus: 9 mg.

180. Lemon Smoothie

PREPARATION TIME
5'

COOK TIME
0'

SERVING
2

INGREDIENTS

- 2 tbsp. lemon juice
- 2 tbsp. brown sugar or stevia
- 4 pasteurized liquid egg whites

DIRECTIONS

1. Combine all ingredients in a blender until smooth.
2. Garnish with a slice of lemon.

NUTRIENTS PER SERVING

- Calories: 49
- Protein: 8 g.
- Fat: 0 g.
- Carb: 5 g.
- Sodium: 110 mg.
- Potassium: 112 mg.
- Phosphorus: 10 mg.

181. Tropical Juice

PREPARATION TIME

5'

COOK TIME

0'

SERVING

2

INGREDIENTS

- 2 cups fresh pineapple, peeled and cut into chunks.
- 1/2 cup low fat coconut milk
- 1 cup of water

DIRECTIONS

1. Add all ingredients to your blender, and blend until smooth.
2. Serve immediately.

Tip: Check with your doctor or dietitian as to whether you can still have coconut milk. Alternatively use non-dairy milk such as almond.

NUTRIENTS PER SERVING

- Calories: 55
- Protein: 7 g.
- Fat: 9 g.
- Carb: 6 g.
- Sodium: 111 mg.
- Potassium: 129 mg.
- Phosphorus: 11 mg.

182. Green Coconut Smoothie

PREPARATION TIME
10'

COOK TIME
3'

SERVING
2

INGREDIENTS

- 1 1/4 cup coconut milk., canned
- 2 tbsp. chia seeds
- 1 cup fresh kale leaves
- 1 cup spinach leaves
- 1 scoop vanilla protein powder
- 1 cup of ice cubes
- Granulated stevia sweetener to taste (optional)
- 1/2 cup water

DIRECTIONS

1. Rinse and clean kale and the spinach leaves from any dirt.
2. Add all ingredients to your blender.
3. Blend until you get a nice smoothie.
4. Serve into chilled glass.

NUTRIENTS PER SERVING

- Calories: 179
- Protein: 4 g.
- Fat: 18 g.
- Carb: 5 g.
- Sodium: 131 mg.
- Potassium: 34 mg.
- Phosphorus: 46 mg.

CHAPTER 25

Special Section 1 - Bread

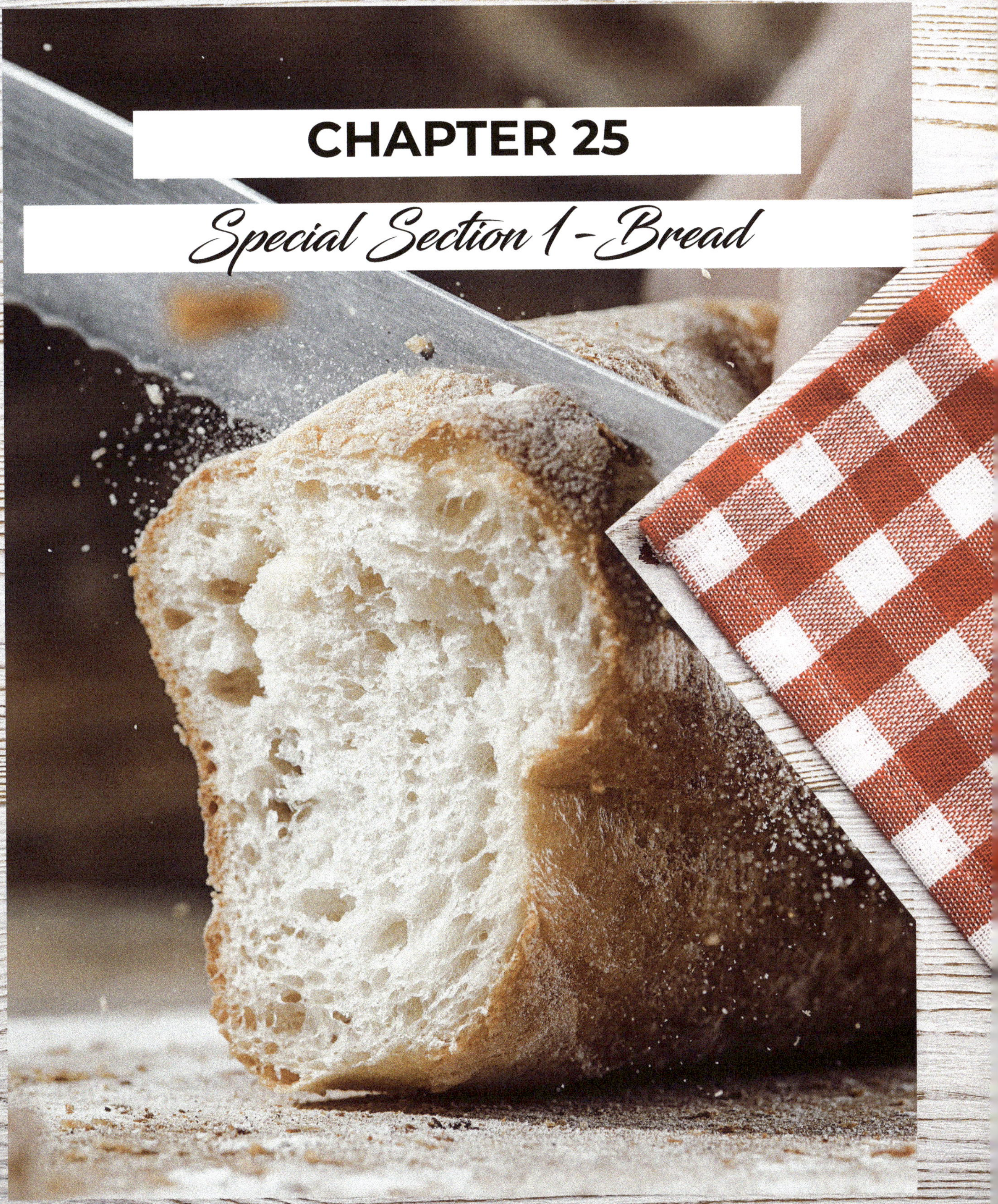

183. Oatmeal Cornbread

PREPARATION TIME
15'

COOK TIME
20'

SERVING
10

INGREDIENTS

- 1 1/2 cups old-fashioned oatmeal
- 1 cup yellow cornmeal
- 1/4 cup granulated sugar
- 2 tsp. baking powder
- 1/4 tsp. salt
- 1 large egg
- 1 cup of soy milk
- 1/2 cup unsweetened applesauce

DIRECTIONS

1. In a food processor, add the oatmeal and pulse until powdered.
2. Transfer the oatmeal powder into a bowl with the cornmeal, sugar, baking powder, and salt, and mix well.
3. Add the egg, soy milk, and applesauce and mix until well combined.
4. Place the mixture into a greased baking pan evenly.
5. Set the cooking time to 20 minutes.
6. Press the "Start/Pause" button to start.
7. When the unit beeps to show that it is preheated, open the lid.
8. Arrange the pan in "Air Fry Basket" and insert it in the oven.
9. Place the pan onto a wire rack for about 10–15 minutes.
10. Carefully, invert the bread onto a wire rack to cool completely before serving.
11. Cut the bread into desired-sized pieces and serve.

NUTRIENTS PER SERVING

- Calories: 136
- Protein: 4.1 g.
- Fat: 2.2 g.
- Carb: 26 g.
- Sodium: 84 mg.
- Potassium: 227 mg.
- Phosphorus: 316 mg.

184. Pineapple Cornbread

PREPARATION TIME
10'

COOK TIME
15'

SERVING
5

INGREDIENTS

- 1 (8 1/2 oz.) package Jiffy corn muffin
- 7 oz. crushed pineapple, canned
- 1/3 cup pineapple juice, canned
- 1 egg

DIRECTIONS

1. In a basin, combine all the ingredients.
2. Place the mixture into the round cake pan.
3. Set the cooking time to 15 minutes.
4. Press the "Start/Pause" button to start.
5. When the unit beeps to show that it is preheated, open the lid.
6. Arrange the pan in "Air Fry Basket" and insert it in the oven.
7. Place the pan onto a wire rack for about 10–15 minutes.
8. Carefully, invert the bread onto a wire rack to cool completely before serving.
9. Cut the bread into desired-sized pieces and serve.

NUTRIENTS PER SERVING

- Calories: 222
- Protein: 3.8 g.
- Fat: 6.4 g.
- Carb: 40.4 g.
- Sodium: 424 mg.
- Potassium: 127 mg.
- Phosphorus: 216 mg.

185. Mini Rosemary Cornbread

PREPARATION TIME
15'

COOK TIME
25'

SERVING
6

INGREDIENTS

- 3/4 cup fine yellow cornmeal
- 1/2 cup sorghum flour
- 1/4 cup tapioca starch
- 1/2 tsp. xanthan gum
- 2 tsp. baking powder
- 1/4 cup granulated sugar
- 1/4 tsp. salt
- 1 cup plain almond milk
- 3 tbsp. olive oil
- 2 tsp. fresh rosemary, minced

DIRECTIONS

1. In a big bowl, mix the flour, cornmeal, starch, sugar, xanthan gum, baking powder, and salt.
2. Add the almond milk, oil, and rosemary. Mix until well combined.
3. Put the mixture into 4 greased ramekins evenly.
4. Set the cooking time to 25 minutes.
5. Press the "Start/Pause" button to start.
6. When the unit beeps to show that it is preheated, open the lid.
7. Arrange the pan in "Air Fry Basket" and insert it in the oven.
8. Place the ramekins onto a wire rack for about 10–15 minutes.
9. Carefully, invert the bread onto a wire rack to cool completely before serving.

NUTRIENTS PER SERVING

- Calories: 220
- Protein: 2.8 g.
- Fat: 8.5 g.
- Carb:35.5 g.
- Sodium: 135 mg.
- Potassium: 327 mg.
- Phosphorus: 216 mg.

186. Monkey Bread

PREPARATION TIME
15'

COOK TIME
7'

SERVING
8

INGREDIENTS

- 1 cup fat-free Greek yogurt
- 1 cup self-rising flour
- 1 tsp. of sugar
- 1/2 tsp. ground cinnamon
- 2 tbsp. butter, melted

DIRECTIONS

1. In a bowl, add the yogurt and flour and mix until a dough comes together.
2. Shape the dough into a ball.
3. Shape the dough ball into a flattened circle.
4. Cut the dough circle into 8 wedges and then, roll each into a ball.
5. In a plastic Ziploc bag, add the sugar, cinnamon, and dough balls.
6. Cover the bag and shake well to coat evenly.
7. Arrange the dough balls in a greased loaf pan.
8. Drizzle the dough balls with butter.
9. Set the cooking time to 7 minutes.
10. Press the "Start/Pause" button to start.
11. When the unit beeps to show that it is preheated, open the lid.
12. Arrange the pan in "Air Fry Basket" and insert it in the oven.
13. Place the pan onto a wire rack for about 5 minutes before serving.

NUTRIENTS PER SERVING

- Calories: 106
- Protein: 3.4 g.
- Fat: 3.4 g.
- Carb: 14.7 g.
- Sodium: 42 mg.
- Potassium: 237 mg.
- Phosphorus: 256 mg.

187. Apple Pull-Apart Bread

PREPARATION TIME
25'

COOK TIME
15'

SERVING
4

INGREDIENTS

- 2 frozen dinner rolls, thawed overnight like Rhodes White Yeast Dinner Rolls
- 1 large Granny Smith apple, sliced, skinned, and chopped
- 1/4 cup brown sugar
- 1/4 cup granulated white sugar
- 4 tsp. ground cinnamon, divided
- 1/4 cup of unsalted butter, melted

DIRECTIONS

1. Cut the dinner rolls in half and then, flatten each into a 2-inch circle.
2. In a large bowl, add the apples, brown sugar, and 2 tsp. of cinnamon and mix well.
3. Place about 1 tsp. of apple mixture filling in the center of each circle.
4. Pinch the edges together to form a smooth ball.
5. Arrange the dough balls in the greased "Air Fry Basket" and insert them in the oven. (Do not turn the oven on.)
6. Let the dough rise for about 1 hour.
7. In a bowl, mix together the white sugar and remaining cinnamon.
8. Remove the basket from the oven and brush the stuffed rolls with butter mixture generously.
9. Sprinkle with the cinnamon sugar on top.
10. Press the "Power" button of the Air Fry Oven and turn the dial to select the "Air Fry" mode.
11. Press the "Time" button and again turn the dial to set the cooking time to 15 minutes.
12. Now push the "Temp" button and rotate the dial to set the temperature at 330°F.
13. Press the "Start/Pause" button to start.
14. When the unit beeps to show that it is preheated, open the lid.
15. Arrange the pan in "Air Fry Basket" and insert it in the oven.
16. Place the pan onto a wire rack for about 5 minutes before serving.

NUTRIENTS PER SERVING

- Calories: 349
- Fat: 14.4 g.
- Carb: 52.8 g.
- Sodium: 315 mg.
- Potassium: 227 mg.
- Phosphorus: 116 mg.

188. Strawberry Bread

PREPARATION TIME
30'

COOK TIME
45'

SERVING
4

INGREDIENTS

- 2 cups fresh strawberries
- 3 1/2 cups all-purpose flour
- 2 cups white sugar
- 1 tbsp. ground cinnamon
- 1 tbsp. salt
- 1 tbsp. baking soda
- 1 1/4 cups vegetable oil
- 4 eggs beaten
- 1 1/4 cups chopped pecans

DIRECTIONS

1. Preheat oven to 350°F. Butter and flour 2 9x5 inch loaf pans.
2. Slice strawberries and place in a medium-sized bowl. Sprinkle lightly with sugar and set aside while preparing batter.
3. Combine flour, sugar, cinnamon, salt, and baking soda in a large bowl, mix well. Blend oil and eggs into strawberries.
4. Add strawberry mixture to flour mixture, blending until dry ingredients are just moistened. Stir in pecans. Divide batter into pans.
5. Bake in the preheated oven until a tester inserted in the center comes out clean. 45–50 minutes later.
6. Let cool in pans on a wire rack for 10 minutes. Turn loaves out of pans and allow to cool before slicing.

NUTRIENTS PER SERVING

- Calories: 281
- Protein 3.3 g.
- Fat: 16.6 g.
- Carb: 31.2 g.
- Sodium: 161.5 mg.
- Potassium: 212 mg.
- Phosphorus: 298 mg.

CHAPTER 26

Special Section 2 - Pasta Salad

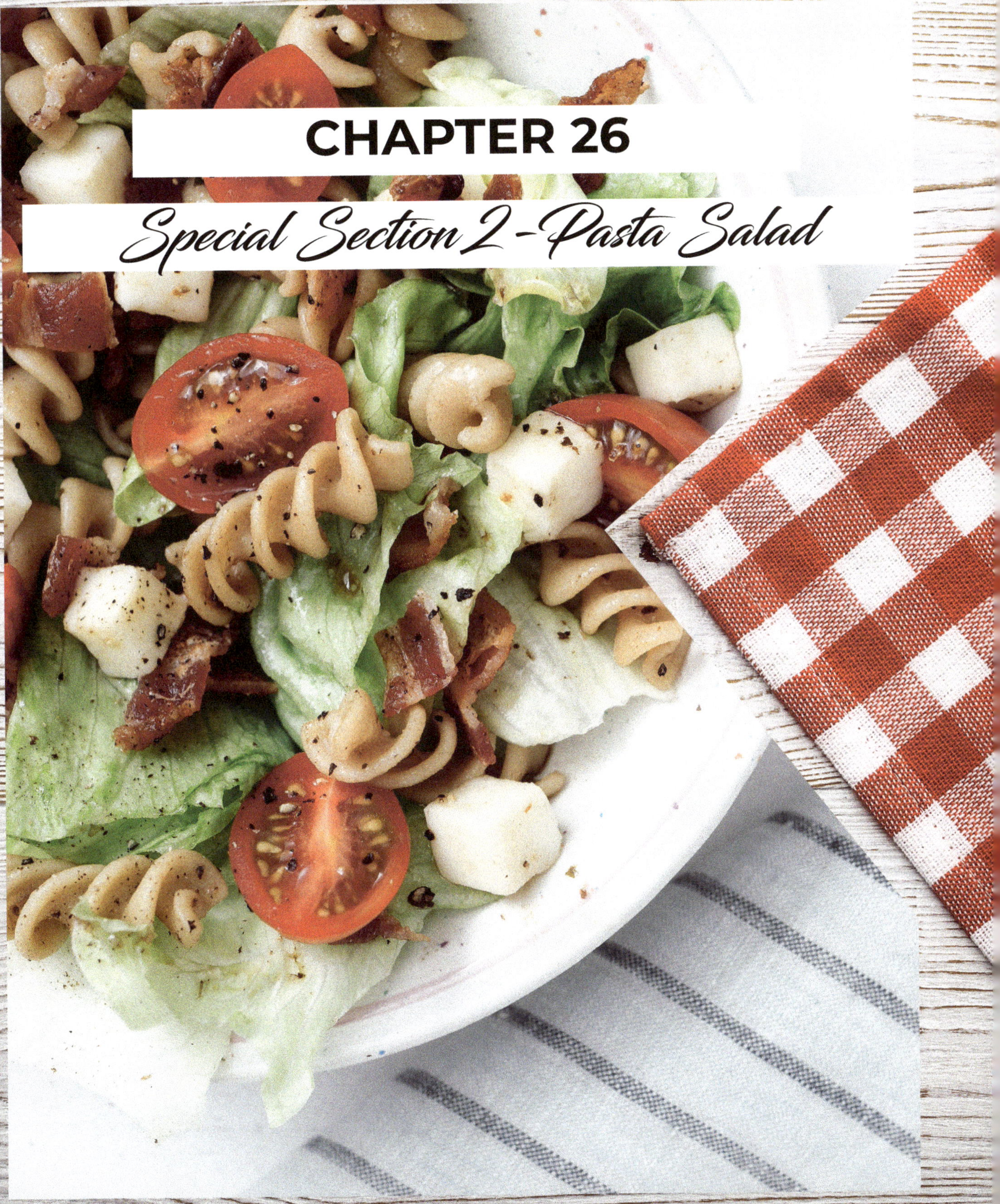

189. Almond Pasta Salad

PREPARATION TIME
10'

COOK TIME
0'

SERVING
14

INGREDIENTS

- 1 lb. elbow macaroni, cooked
- 1/2 cup sun-dried tomatoes, diced
- 1 (15 oz.) can whole artichokes, diced
- 1 orange bell pepper, diced
- 3 green onions, sliced
- 2 tbsp. basil, sliced
- 2 oz. slivered almonds

Dressing:

- 1 garlic clove, minced
- 1 tbsp. Dijon mustard
- 1 tbsp. raw honey
- 1/4 cup white balsamic vinegar
- 1/3 cup olive oil

DIRECTIONS

1. Take a suitable salad bowl.
2. Start tossing in all the ingredients.
3. Mix well and serve.

NUTRIENTS PER SERVING

- Calories: 260
- Protein: 9.6 g.
- Fat: 7.7 g.
- Carb: 41.4 g.
- Sodium: 143 mg.
- Potassium: 585 mg.
- Phosphorus: 39 mg.

190. Zucchini Pasta With Mango-Kiwi Sauce

PREPARATION TIME
5'

COOK TIME
20'

SERVING
2

INGREDIENTS

- 1 tsp. dried herbs (optional)
- 1/2 cup raw kale leaves, shredded
- 2 small dried figs
- 3 Medjool dates
- 4 medium kiwis
- 2 large mangos, seed discarded
- 2 cup zucchini, spiralized
- 1/4 cup roasted cashew

DIRECTIONS

1. On a salad bowl, place kale then topped with zucchini noodles and sprinkle with dried herbs. Set aside.
2. In a food processor, grind to a powder the cashews. Add figs, dates, kiwis, and mangoes then puree to a smooth consistency.
3. Pour over zucchini pasta, serve, and enjoy.

NUTRIENTS PER SERVING

- Calories: 530
- Protein: 8 g.
- Fat: 18.5 g.
- Carb: 95.4 g.
- Sodium: 161 mg.
- Potassium: 227 mg.
- Phosphorus: 316 mg.

191. Baked Portobello, Pasta 'n Cheese

PREPARATION TIME
10'

COOK TIME
30'

SERVING
4

INGREDIENTS

- 1 cup milk
- 1 cup mozzarella cheese, shredded
- 1 large clove garlic, minced
- 1 tbsp. vegetable oil
- 1/4 cup margarine
- 1/4 tsp. dried basil
- 1/4 lb. Portobello mushrooms, thinly sliced
- 2 tbsp. all-purpose flour
- 2 tbsp. soy sauce
- 4 oz. penne pasta, cooked according to manufacturer's Directions for Cooking
- 5 oz. frozen spinach, chopped, thawed

DIRECTIONS

1. Lightly grease the baking pan of the air fryer with oil. For 2 minutes, heat on 360°F. Add mushrooms and cook for a minute. Transfer to a plate.
2. In the same pan, melt margarine for a minute. Stir in basil, garlic, and flour. Cook for 3 minutes. Stir and cook for another 2 minutes. Stir in half of the milk slowly while whisking continuously. Cook for another 2 minutes. Mix well. Cook for another 2 minutes. Stir in remaining milk and cook for another 3 minutes.
3. Add cheese and mix well.
4. Stir in soy sauce, spinach, mushrooms, and pasta. Mix well. Top with remaining cheese.
5. Cook for 15 minutes at 390°F until tops are lightly browned.
6. Serve and enjoy.

NUTRIENTS PER SERVING

- Calories: 482
- Protein: 16.0 g.
- Fat: 32.1 g.
- Carb: 32.1 g.
- Sodium: 131 mg.
- Potassium: 297 mg.
- Phosphorus: 236 mg.

192. Zucchini Pasta

PREPARATION TIME
15'

COOK TIME
30'

SERVING
4

INGREDIENTS

- 8 oz. farfalle pasta, uncooked
- 3 tbsp. olive oil
- 2 garlic cloves, minced
- 3 large zucchinis, diced
- Sea salt and black pepper to taste
- 1/2 cup milk, 2%
- 1/4 tsp. nutmeg
- 1 tbsp. lemon juice, fresh
- 1/2 cup Parmesan cheese, grated

DIRECTIONS

1. Get out a skillet and place it over medium heat, and then heat up the oil. Add in your garlic and cook for a minute. Stir often so that it doesn't burn.
2. Add in your salt, pepper, and zucchini. Stir well, and cook covered for 15 minutes. During this time, you'll want to stir the mixture twice.
3. Get out a microwave-safe bowl, and heat the milk for 30 seconds. Stir in your nutmeg, and then pour it into the skillet.
4. Cook uncovered for 5 minutes. Stir occasionally to keep from burning.
5. Get out a stockpot and cook your pasta per package instructions. Drain the pasta, and then save 2 tbsp. of pasta water.
6. Stir everything together, and add the cheese, lemon juice, and pasta water.

NUTRIENTS PER SERVING

- Calories: 410
- Protein: 15 g.
- Fat: 17 g.
- Carb: 45 g.
- Sodium: 127 mg.
- Potassium: 227 mg.
- Phosphorus: 316 mg.

193. Asparagus Pasta

PREPARATION TIME
10'

COOK TIME
25'

SERVING
6

INGREDIENTS

- 8 oz. farfalle pasta, uncooked
- 1 1/2 cups asparagus, fresh, trimmed, chopped into 1-inch pieces
- 1-pint grape tomatoes, halved
- 2 tbsp. olive oil
- Sea salt and black pepper to taste
- 2 cups mozzarella, fresh, drained
- 1/3 cup basil leaves, fresh, torn
- 2 tbsp. balsamic vinegar

DIRECTIONS

1. Start by heating the oven to 400°F, and then get out a stockpot. Cook your pasta per package instructions, and reserve 1/4 cup of pasta water.
2. Get out a bowl and toss the tomatoes, oil, asparagus, and season with salt and pepper.
3. Spread this mixture on a baking sheet, and bake for fifteen minutes. Stir twice this time.
4. Remove your vegetables from the oven, and then add the cooked pasta to your baking sheet.
5. Mix with a few tbsp. of pasta water so that your sauce becomes smoother.
6. Mix in your basil and mozzarella, drizzling with balsamic vinegar. Serve warm.

NUTRIENTS PER SERVING

- Calories: 307
- Protein: 18 g.
- Fat: 14 g.
- Carb: 33 g.
- Sodium: 141 mg.
- Potassium: 227 mg.
- Phosphorus: 316 mg.

194. Pasta Pesto Salad

PREPARATION TIME
15'

COOK TIME
15'

SERVING
4

INGREDIENTS

- 12 oz. whole-wheat rotini pasta
- 1 cup fresh basil leaves
- 1/2 cup packed fresh flat-leaf parsley leaves
- 1/2 cup arugula, chopped
- 2 tbsp. Parmesan cheese, grated
- 1/4 cup extra-virgin olive oil
- 3 tbsp. mayonnaise
- 2 tbsp. water
- 1 red bell pepper, chopped
- 1 medium yellow summer squash, sliced
- 1 cup frozen baby peas, softened and drained

DIRECTIONS

1. Boil water in a big pot.
2. Meanwhile, combine the basil, parsley, arugula, cheese, and olive oil in a blender or food processor.
3. Blend or process until the herbs are finely chopped. Add the mayonnaise and water, then process again. Set aside.
4. Put the pasta in the pot of boiling water; cook according to package directions, about 8–9 minutes.
5. Drain well, reserving 1/4 cup of the cooking liquid.
6. Combine the pesto, pasta, bell pepper, squash, and peas in a large bowl and toss gently, adding enough of the reserved pasta cooking liquid to make a sauce on the salad.
7. Serve immediately or cover and chill, then serve.
8. Store covered in the refrigerator for up to 3 days.

NUTRIENTS PER SERVING

- Calories: 378
- Protein: 9 g.
- Fat: 24 g.
- Carb: 35 g.
- Sodium: 163 mg.
- Potassium: 472 mg.
- Phosphorus: 213 mg.

CHAPTER 27

Special Section 3 - Extra Yummy Meals

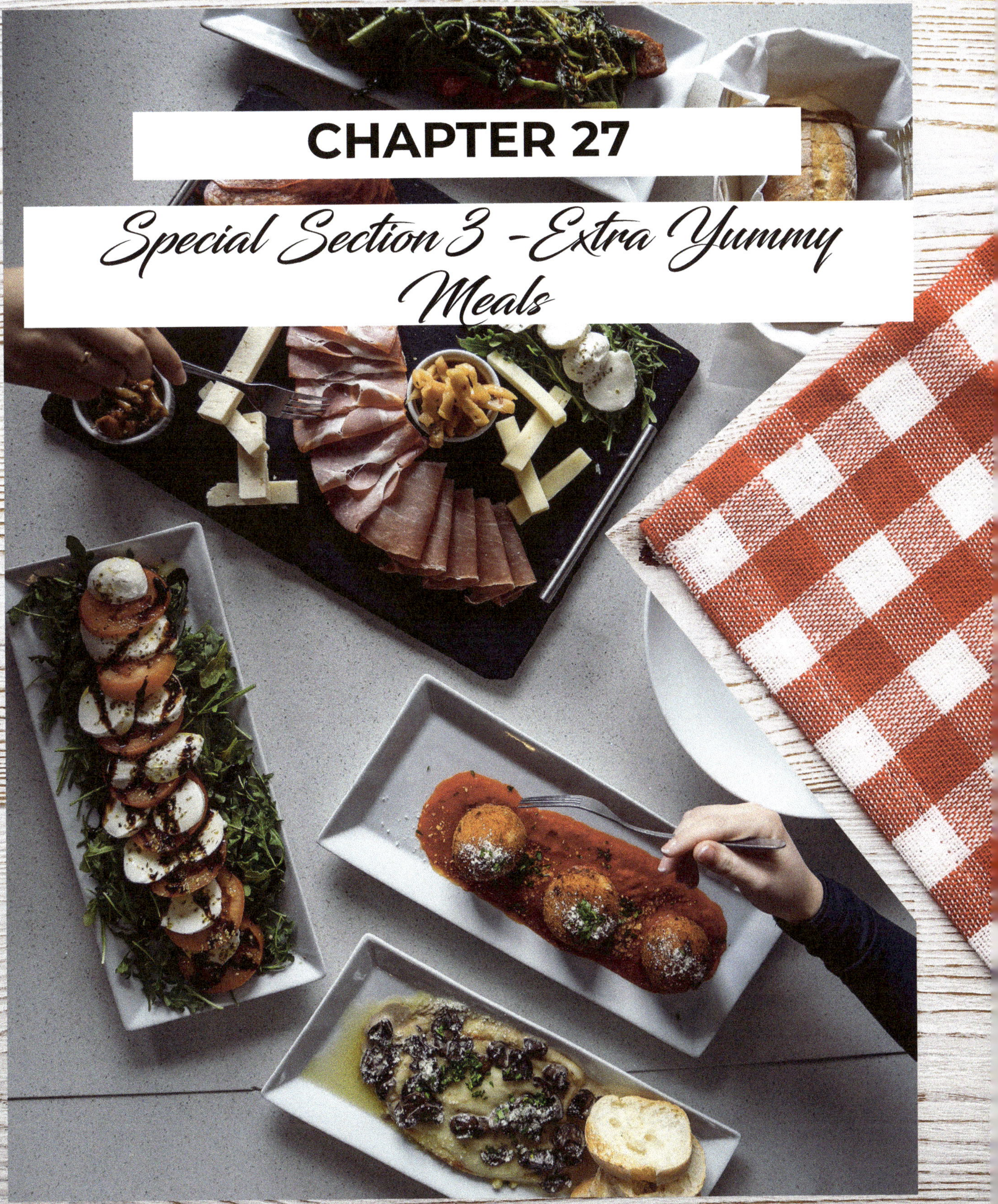

195. Apple Spice Pork Chops

PREPARATION TIME

10'

COOK TIME

10'

SERVING

4

INGREDIENTS

- 2 medium apples: peeled, cored, sliced
- 1 lb. pork chops
- 1/4 tsp. salt
- 1/4 cup brown sugar
- 1/4 tsp. ground nutmeg
- 1/4 tsp. ground black pepper
- 1/4 tsp. cinnamon
- 2 tbsp. unsalted butter

DIRECTIONS

1. Switch on the broiler, let it preheat, then place pork chops in it and cook for 5 minutes per side until done.
2. Meanwhile, take a medium-sized skillet pan, place it over medium heat, add butter and when it melts, add apples, sprinkle with black pepper, salt, sugar, cinnamon, and nutmeg, stir well and cook for 8 minutes, or until apples are tender and the sauce has thickened to the desired level.
3. When done, spoon the applesauce over pork chops and serve.

NUTRIENTS PER SERVING

- Calories: 306
- Protein: 22 g.
- Fat: 16 g.
- Carb: 21 g.
- Sodium: 192 mg.
- Potassium: 227 mg.
- Phosphorus: 316 mg.

196. Beef Burritos

PREPARATION TIME
10'

COOK TIME
20'

SERVING
6

INGREDIENTS

- 1/4 cup white onion, chopped
- 1/4 cup green bell pepper, chopped
- 1 lb. ground beef
- 1/4 cup tomato puree, low sodium
- 1/4 tsp. ground black pepper
- 1/4 tsp. ground cumin
- 6 flour tortillas, burrito size

DIRECTIONS

1. Take a skillet pan, place it over medium heat and, when hot, add beef and cook for 5–8 minutes until browned.
2. Drain the excess fat, then transfer beef to a plate lined with paper towels and serve.
3. Return pan over medium heat, grease it with oil and when hot, add pepper and onion and cook for 5 minutes, or until softened.
4. Switch to low heat, return beef to the pan, season with black pepper and cumin, pour in tomato puree, stir until mixed and cook for 5 minutes until done.
5. Dispense beef combination evenly on top of the tortilla, roll them in burrito style by folding both ends, and then serve.

NUTRIENTS PER SERVING

- Calories: 265
- Protein: 15 g.
- Fat: 9 g.
- Carb: 31 g.
- Sodium: 341 mg.
- Potassium: 127 mg.
- Phosphorus: 286 mg.

197. Broccoli and Beef Stir-Fry

PREPARATION TIME
5'

COOK TIME
20'

SERVING
4

INGREDIENTS

- 12 oz. frozen broccoli, thawed
- 8 oz. sirloin beef, cut into thin strips
- 1 medium Roma tomato, chopped
- 1 tsp. garlic, minced
- 1 tbsp. cornstarch
- 2 tbsp. soy sauce, reduced-sodium
- 1/4 cup chicken broth, low sodium
- 2 tbsp. peanut oil
- 2 cups cooked brown rice

DIRECTIONS

1. Take a frying pan, place it over medium heat, add oil and when hot, add garlic and cook for 1 minute until fragrant.
2. Add vegetable blend, cook for 5 minutes, then transfer vegetable blend to a plate and set aside until needed.
3. Add beef strips into the pan, and then cook for 7 minutes until cooked to the desired level.
4. Prepare the sauce by putting cornstarch in a bowl, and then whisking in soy sauce and broth until well combined.
5. Returned vegetables to the pan, add tomatoes, drizzle with sauce, stir well until coated, and cook for 2 minutes until the sauce has thickened.
6. Serve with brown rice.

NUTRIENTS PER SERVING

- Calories: 373
- Protein: 18 g.
- Fat: 17 g.
- Carb: 37 g.
- Sodium: 351 mg.
- Potassium: 236 mg.
- Phosphorus: 236 mg.

198. Swiss Seafood Canapés

PREPARATION TIME
20'

COOK TIME
25'

SERVING
4

INGREDIENTS

- 1 can (6 oz.) small shrimp, rinsed and drained
- 1 package (6 oz.) frozen crabmeat, thawed
- 1 cup Swiss cheese, shredded
- 2 large eggs, hard-boiled, chopped
- 1/4 cup finely chopped celery
- 1/4 cup mayonnaise
- 1/4 cup French salad dressing or seafood cocktail sauce
- 2 green onions, chopped
- Dash salt
- 1 loaf (16 oz.) snack rye bread

DIRECTIONS

1. Add the first 9 ingredients to a large container. Put bread on ungreased baking sheets.
2. Broil for 1–2 minutes, 4–6-inches from the heat, or until lightly browned. Flip slices over; spread 1 rounded tbsp. full of seafood mixture on each.
3. Broil for 4–5 more minutes or until heated through.

NUTRIENTS PER SERVING

- Calories: 57
- Protein: 3 g.
- Fat: 3 g.
- Carb: 5 g.
- Sodium: 156 mg.
- Potassium: 327 mg.
- Phosphorus: 316 mg.

199. Ground Beef and Rice Soup

PREPARATION TIME
15'

COOK TIME
40'

SERVING
4

INGREDIENTS

- 1/2 lb ground beef, extra-lean
- 1/2 small sweet onion, chopped
- 1 tsp. garlic, minced
- 2 cups of water
- 1 cup beef broth, low-sodium
- 1/2 cup long-grain white rice, uncooked
- 1 celery stalk, chopped
- 1/2 cup fresh green beans, cut into 1-inch pieces
- 1 tsp. fresh thyme, chopped
- Ground black pepper to taste

DIRECTIONS

1. Sauté the ground beef in a saucepan for 6 minutes or until the beef is completely browned.
2. Drain off the excess fat and add the onion and garlic to the saucepan.
3. Sauté the vegetables for about 3 minutes, or until they are softened.
4. Add the celery, rice, beef broth, and water.
5. Boil the soup, reduce the heat to low, and simmer for 30 minutes or until the rice is tender.
6. Add the green beans and thyme and simmer for 3 minutes.
7. Remove the soup from the heat and season with pepper.

NUTRIENTS PER SERVING

- Calories: 154
- Protein: 9 g.
- Fat: 7 g.
- Carb: 14 g.
- Sodium: 133 mg.
- Potassium: 227 mg.
- Phosphorus: 316 mg.

200. Shrimp With Dipping Sauce

PREPARATION TIME
5'

COOK TIME
15'

SERVING
6

INGREDIENTS

- 1 tbsp. soy sauce, reduced-sodium
- 2 tsp. hot pepper sauce
- 1 tsp. canola oil
- 1/4 tsp. garlic powder
- 1/8 –1/4 tsp. cayenne pepper
- 1 lb. medium shrimp, uncooked, peeled, and deveined
- 2 tbsp. green onions, chopped

Dipping sauce:

- 3 tbsp. soy sauce, reduced-sodium
- 1 tsp. rice vinegar
- 1 tbsp. orange juice
- 2 tsp. sesame oil
- 2 tsp. honey
- 1 garlic clove, minced
- 1 1/2 tsp. fresh ginger root, minced

DIRECTIONS

1. Heat the initial 5 ingredients in a big nonstick frying pan for 30 seconds, then mix continuously.
2. Add onions and shrimp and stir fry for 4–5 minutes or until the shrimp turns pink. Mix together the sauce ingredients and serve it with the shrimp.

NUTRIENTS PER SERVING

- Calories: 97
- Protein: 13 g.
- Fat: 3 g.
- Carb: 4 g.
- Sodium: 143 mg.
- Potassium: 297 mg.
- Phosphorus: 196 mg.

201. Seafood Casserole

PREPARATION TIME
20'

COOK TIME
45'

SERVING
4

INGREDIENTS

- 2 cups eggplant, peeled and diced into 1-inch pieces
- Butter, for greasing the baking dish
- 1 tbsp. olive oil
- 1/2 sweet onion, chopped
- 1 tsp. garlic, minced
- 1 celery stalk, chopped
- 1/2 red bell pepper, boiled and chopped
- 3 tbsp. lemon juice, freshly squeezed
- 1 tsp. hot sauce
- 1/4 tsp. creole seasoning mix
- 1/2 cup white rice, uncooked
- 1 large egg
- 4 oz. shrimp, cooked
- 6 oz. queen crab meat

DIRECTIONS

1. Preheat the oven to 350°F.
2. Boil the eggplant in a saucepan for 5 minutes. Drain and set aside.
3. Grease a 9x13-inch baking dish with butter and set aside.
4. Heat the olive oil in a large skillet over medium heat.
5. Sauté the garlic, onion, celery, and bell pepper for 4 minutes or until tender.
6. Add the sautéed vegetables to the eggplant, along with the lemon juice, hot sauce, seasoning, rice, and egg.
7. Stir to combine.
8. Fold in the shrimp and crab meat.
9. Spoon the casserole mixture into the casserole dish, patting down the top.
10. Bake for 25–30 minutes or until casserole is heated through and rice is tender.
11. Serve warm.

- NUTRIENTS PER SERVING
- Calories: 118
- Protein: 12 g.
- Fat: 4 g.
- Carb: 9 g.
- Sodium: 235 mg.
- Potassium: 199 mg.
- Phosphorus: 102 mg.

PART 3

Measurement Conversions

	US STANDARD	US STANDARD (OZ.)	METRIC (APPROXIMATE)		
VOLUME EQUIVALENTS (LIQUID)	2 tbsp.	1 fl. oz.	30 ml.		
	1/4 cup	2 fl. oz.	60 ml.		
	1/2 cup	4 fl. oz.	120 ml.		
	1 cup	8 fl. oz.	240 ml.		
	11/2 cups	12 fl. oz.	355 ml.		
	2 cups or 1 pint	16 fl. oz.	475 ml.		
	4 cups or 1 1/4	32 fl. oz.	1 l.		
	1 gallon	128 fl. oz.	4 l.		
	VOLUME EQUIVALENTS (DRY)	1/8 tsp.	________	0.5 ml.	
		1/4 tsp.	________	1 ml.	
		1/2 tsp.	________	2 ml.	
		3/4 tsp.	________	4 ml.	
		1 tsp.	________	5 ml.	
		1 tbsp.	________	15 ml.	
		1/4 cup	________	59 ml.	
		1/3 cup	________	79 ml.	
		1/2 cup	________	118 ml.	
		2/3 cup	________	156 ml.	
		3/4 cup	________	177 ml.	
		1 cup	________	235 ml.	
		2 cups or 1 pint	________	475 ml.	

		3 cups	________	700 ml.	
		4 cups or 1 1/4	________	1 l.	
		1/2 gallon	________	2 l.	
		1 gallon	________	4 l.	
		WEIGHT EQUIVALENTS	1/2 oz	________	15 g
			1 oz.	________	30 g
			2 oz	________	60 g
			4 oz.	________	115 g
			8 oz.	________	225 g
			12 oz	________	340 g
			16 oz. or 1 lb.	________	455 g

	FAHRENHEIT (F)	CELSIUS (C) (APPROXIMATE)
OVEN TEMPERATURES	250°F	120°C
	300°F	150°C
	325°F	180°C
	375°F	190°C
	400°F	200°C
	425°F	220°C
	450°F	230°C

CONCLUSION

You likely had little knowledge about your kidneys before. You probably didn't know how you could take steps to improve your kidney health and decrease the risk of developing kidney failure. However, through reading this book, you now understand the power of the human kidney, as well as the prognosis of chronic kidney disease. While over 30 million Americans are being affected by kidney disease, you can now take steps to be one of the people who is actively working to promote your kidney health. Kidney disease now ranks as the 18th deadliest condition in the world. In the United States alone, it is reported that over 600,000 Americans succumb to kidney failure.

These stats are alarming, which is why, it is necessary to take proper care of your kidneys, starting with a kidney-friendly diet. These recipes are ideal whether you have been diagnosed with a kidney problem or you want to prevent any kidney issue.

With regards to your wellbeing and health, it's a smart thought to see your doctor as frequently as conceivable to ensure you don't run into preventable issues that you needn't get. The kidneys are your body's toxin channel (just like the liver), cleaning the blood of remote substances and toxins that are discharged from things like preservatives in the food and other toxins. Your kidneys are working to clean your body when you eat flippantly and fill your body with toxins, either from nourishment, when you drink (liquor or alcohol for instance), or even from the air you inhale (free radicals are in the sun and move through your skin, through messy air, and numerous food sources contain them). Your body additionally will in general convert numerous things that appear to be benign until your body's organs convert them into things like formaldehyde because of a synthetic response and transforming phase.

One case of this is a large portion of those diet sugars utilized in diet soft drinks, for instance, Aspartame transforms into formaldehyde in the body. These toxins must be expelled, or they can prompt ailment, renal (kidney) failure, malignant growth, and several painful problems.

This isn't a condition that occurs without any forethought, it is a dynamic issue, and may be both found early and treated, diet changed, and settling what is causing the condition. It's conceivable to have partial renal failure yet, as a rule; it requires some time (or downright awful diet for a short time) to arrive at absolute renal failure. You would prefer not to reach total renal failure since this will require standard dialysis treatments to save your life. Dialysis treatments explicitly clean the blood of waste and toxins in the blood utilizing a machine because your body can no longer carry out the responsibility. Without treatments, you could die a very painful death. Renal failure can be the consequence of long-haul diabetes, hypertension, unreliable diet, and can stem from other health concerns.

A renal diet is tied in with directing the intake of protein and phosphorus in your eating routine. Restricting your sodium intake is likewise significant. By controlling these 2 variables you can control the vast majority of the toxins/waste made by your body and, thus, this enables your kidney to 100% function. In the event that you get this early enough and truly moderate your diets with extraordinary consideration, you could avert all-out renal failure. As you get this early, you can take out the issue completely.

Lightning Source UK Ltd.
Milton Keynes UK
UKHW050858070121
376584UK00003B/26

9 781801 135863